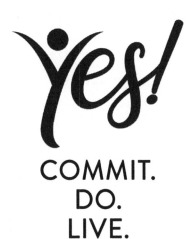

COMMIT.
DO.
LIVE.

Embrace the Brain-Body Connection
to Achieve Your True Desires

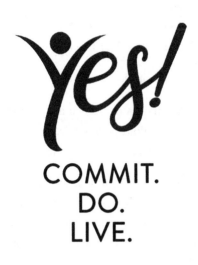

COMMIT.
DO.
LIVE.

*Embrace the Brain-Body Connection
to Achieve Your True Desires*

LISA CHARLES

Niche Pressworks

YES! COMMIT. DO. LIVE.
Embrace the Brain-Body Connection to Achieve Your True Desires

ISBN-13:   978-1-952654-31-2 (Paperback)
            978-1-952654-32-9 (eBook)
            978-1-952654-99-2 (Hardback)

The information provided in this guide is for educational purposes only. I am not a doctor, and this is not meant to be taken as medical advice. The information provided in this guide is based upon my experiences, as well as our interpretations of the current research available.

The advice and tips given in this book are meant for healthy adults only. You should consult your physician to ensure tips given in this book are appropriate for your individual circumstances.

If you have any health issues or pre-existing conditions, please consult with your physician before implementing any of the information provided herein.

This book is for informational purposes only and the author does not accept any responsibilities for any liabilities or damages, real or perceived, resulting from the use of this information.

For permission to reprint portions of this content or bulk purchases, contact YES! Coach Lisa at www.YesCoachLisa.com

Published by Niche Pressworks: http://NichePressworks.com

Illustrations by: Alexey Leo Tkachenko
Cover Photo: Jeffrey Hornstein, Photographer

DEDICATION

I dedicate this book to my loving and support-ive parents, Laverne Millicent Russell and Edgar Russell Jr. I have been abundantly blessed to have a mother and father who are both incredible role models 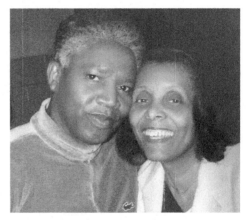 and have always been a great source of encouragement through-out all my life endeavors.

They helped to plant the seeds from which this book has grown.

My mother, a high school debate champion and Howard University Thespian, dedicated her life to enriching and trans-forming the lives of our youth through her lifelong commitment as a social worker.

My father, a U.S. Air Force Korean War veteran and journal-ism graduate of Duquesne University, spent many of his profes-sional work years as a writer and communications manager for I.B.M. and a marketing director for United Way.

Both of my parents were trailblazers within their professions, often integrating their work environments while advancing based upon their skill, dedication, and passion.

How fortunate I am to have been blessed with both of them, and I thank them for being my inspiration!

CONTENTS

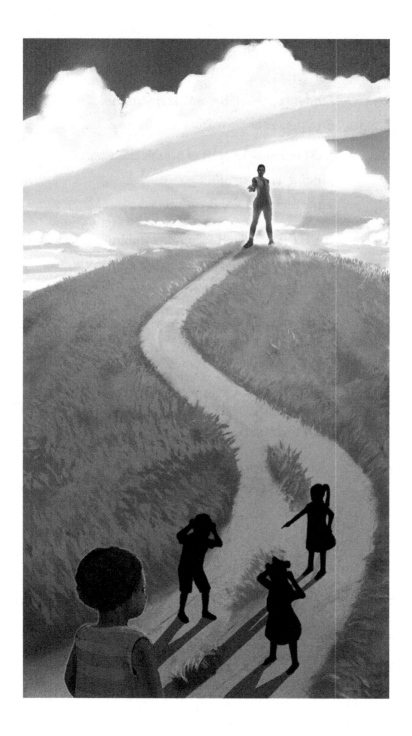

CHAPTER 1

KNOW YOUR TRUTH—
MY SECRET PAIN REVEALED

*"There is no greater agony than bearing
an untold story inside you."*
—MAYA ANGELOU

The Mack—Life Begins

Growing up in the suburbs of Maryland, I was a chunky child. I had one of those little potbellies that showed prominently in my clothing—winter, spring, summer, and fall.

Funny, but early on, my size never really bothered me or had any effect on my behavior. It didn't prevent me from joining the town's swim team, nor did it prevent me from enjoying neighborhood play with the assortment of children that lived on our block. I didn't really focus on or define myself by my weight until one day I realized how others did.

I had this nickname— "MACK." When it was time for all of us to meet after school in the street to decide what games we would play, I would run down the hill, and a group of neighbors would all scream with absolute enthusiasm, "MACK! MACK! MACK!"

I loved it! I mean, I really loved it! I would have such a goofy smile on my face. I felt many of the universal desires—to be popular, accepted, and loved.

I held tightly to that feeling until one day while driving with my parents on a highway, I noticed the prominent print on the front of a massive semi-truck: "MACK." Once I saw one truck, it was as if I had seen all trucks. At that moment, my perspective completely changed.

In the blink of an eye, I realized that during all those years, my neighborhood friends had been calling me fat. Instead of supporting me as friends, they saw me as a massive truck. That insult cut painfully deeply and left a lasting wound. I was sad, ashamed, rejected, defeated, and full of self-doubt. In that one moment, I saw everything through the prism of weight, and weight became a driving issue in my life.

For the next thirty years, weight would dictate the diets I chose, the extreme fitness I attempted, the way I believed people perceived me, and most importantly, the way I perceived myself. In many ways, I gave weight power and dominion over me, and in some cases, it clouded my vision of my true desires. Weight held a place of importance until I learned how to take my power back.

Forget "Sticks and stones will break your bones, but names will never hurt you." Words are powerful. Words can destroy.

We know that science puts great importance on the power that words, both positive and negative, can have on the brain. Words help to create thoughts, which can lead to action, either good or bad. When those words become self-talk, they can lead to long-term harm.

Science Speaks

According to scientific studies, positive and negative words affect us on a *deep psychological level* and significantly impact the outcome of our lives.[1] Negative, painful words, whether spoken or heard, lead to "activations within regions of the pain matrix" in the brain.[2]

Essentially, negative words release stress and anxiety-inducing hormones in subjects. However, I could bury that pain deep inside—so deep that I could pretend it did not even exist. Or so I thought.

---

1   Maria Richter, Judith Eck, Thomas Straube, Wolfgang H.R. Miltner, and Thomas Weiss, "Do words hurt? Brain activation during the processing of pain-related words." *Pain:* February 2010 148(2), 204.

2   Lindsey Horton, "The Neuroscience Behind Our Words," Business Relationship Management Institute, August 8, 2019, https://brm.institute/neuroscience-behind-words/.

The Power of Pain

"We must embrace pain and burn it as fuel for our journey."
—KENJI MIYAZAWA

Though I didn't know it, my pain took up residence inside me. It gained a semi-permanent home from which it could influence my behavior, engender unhealthy habits, and create negative thoughts designed to enslave my mind and body. The funny thing about pain, whether acknowledged or not, is that it can control behavior and disrupt the achievement of any desire.

During my thirty-year hiatus from living a life of lasting health and wellness, my pain lead me down the dangerous path of a Yo-Yo dieter. This path of ongoing cycles of weight loss and weight gain has a detrimental impact on the body, from disrupting hormonal balance to increasing the risk of heart disease, diabetes, high blood pressure, and premature death.[3] The risks were real, but I didn't know about them in my early life, and I unwittingly walked a path that imperiled my health.

My journey as a Yo-Yo'er began shortly after the MACK incident. At the age of eleven, my sister and I embarked on the "Banana Diet." We survived on three bananas, a gallon of water, and intense daily physical exercise each day for seven days. Both my sister and I developed an unhealthy relationship with food

---

3   Tae Jung Oh, Jae Hoon Moon, Sung Hee Choi, Soo Lim, Kyong Soo Park, Nam H Cho, and Hak Chul Jang. "Body-Weight Fluctuation and Incident Diabetes Mellitus, Cardiovascular Disease, and Mortality: A 16-Year Prospective Cohort Study." The Journal of Clinical Endocrinology & Metabolism 104, no. 3 (March 1, 2019): 644. https://doi.org/10.1210/jc.2018-01239.

and movement. We operated on the extreme, and the Banana Diet was just the beginning.

I was desperate to change my body, and that desperation pushed me through that crazy diet. Surprise! *(not)*—we lost weight, and everyone commented how good we looked, even though I had more pounds to lose. For me, at that time, the jury was in.

If you lose weight—no matter the emotional or health costs— people will love and accept you.

That was a dangerous message then, and it is a dangerous message now—but it is one that many of us live by and don't even know it.

As with most diets, success is often short-lived, and the Banana Diet was no exception. Over the years, it was followed by an assortment of fad diets we found in books and magazines or learned about from friends or established diet centers. I followed various meal plans and "no eating" challenges. The unhealthy Yo-Yo rhythm that developed played as a negative thought loop through my life.

First, I would get disgusted and disappointed with myself. Maybe I did not fit into a certain outfit or did not like the glimpse of my true self I caught in a mirror. *(Damn those mall mirrors.)* The most vile, negative self-talk would begin. "How did you let this happen?" "What is wrong with you?" "Don't you have will-power?" "You always fail."

I, like other Yo-Yo'ers, would then embark on some type of deprivation eating plan, from starvation to one from the many weight-loss centers that boldly advertised the "dream body" or the "quick fix." Liquid diets, magazine diets, anything was possible. However, regardless of the path the Yo-Yo'er takes, the end is always the same—all roads lead to failure until you commit to making a change from within. And that commitment doesn't come with a quick fix.

I would experience various levels of "success" until I would give up and return to the old habits that comforted me but did not serve me. Each failure, whether I admitted to it or not, chipped away at my vision for the future. Each failure reenforced a variety of bad habits: avoidance, denial, lies, overeating, undereating, and secret eating. And, sadly, each failure reenforced my loss of personal power. That's the Yo-Yo life— destructive to brain, body, spirit, and the belief that change is truly possible.

Throughout my various career paths as a state and federal prosecutor, an actress, a singer, and a speaker, I stayed on the Yo-Yo plan. I was able to compartmentalize this area of my life, creating a false belief that I had it all under control. After all, if I could accomplish the roles and responsibilities that my career path demanded of me, certainly I could control my weight.

I learned how wrong I was when my Yo-Yo lifestyle began to impact my health. My "Ah-Ha" moment came after years of dieting and multiple years of inconsistent bouts of extreme exercise. That moment literally stopped me in my tracks, changed my thinking about health, and led me to a path that altered almost every aspect of my life.

My "Ah-Ha" Moment

"One thing you can't hide is when you're crippled inside."
—JOHN LENNON

One day, I found myself lying on my back, looking up at a slightly buzzing fluorescent ceiling light in a white, sterile hospital room. A curtain enclosed my bed, and I was hooked up to an IV, in pain, suffering with an intestinal illness. Earlier that day, I had received news that rivaled my physical pain and made me face my truth. When I was weighed by hospital staff, I found out that I was forty-five pounds heavier than I thought possible. That was forty-five pounds on top of what I already thought was a heavy weight. It was so depressing and overwhelming. Through years of gaining and losing weight and exercising and not exercising, I had lost muscle, gained fat, and now had trouble digesting a variety of foods and sleeping through the night. I felt so tired and lethargic.

I was a mess!

It was a moment of personal reckoning. The truth was in—I had let myself go to a place that I now found completely unrecognizable, and there was no more hiding or pretending. I remember crying that inconsolable cry, feeling so sorry for myself.

But then, I realized that now was the time for me to get control over my body. That had been the one area of my life in which I had never experienced sustained success.

By that point, I was a lifetime member of two diet centers (*one could ask why they have lifetime memberships*) and was an expert Yo-Yo'er.

But now, I was ready to say, "*I will diet NO MORE.*"

I committed myself to finding a healthy way to transform myself from the inside out through exploration of the way the brain and body work together—the "brain-body connection." I knew if I was going to bring about lasting change, I could not focus on just fitness nor just food. I had to commit to understanding my whole self, and I was ready to figure out how to experience sustained and substantial change.

Diet No More

"Failure gave me strength. Pain was my motivation."
—MICHAEL JORDAN

Where to begin?

I had to begin at the origin of my poor decision-making. For me, a lot rested in my MACK moment. I had to shine a light on that pain and identify all of the mental, physical, and emotional habits that sprang from it and also kept it in power over the years. By allowing myself to go where I did not wish to venture, I stripped the MACK moment of its dominion over me and my decisions moving forward. It was the beginning of my YES! Mindset transformative journey.

All of the failure, disappointment, anger, and fear of the future showed themselves in the stuff I harbored in my home. I had a giant pile of useless products, vitamins, strange equipment, braces, magnets, tapes, CDs, gadgets, books and magazines, and cut-out articles, all representing the promise of change that I never fully realized.

> Out with the old way, and in with the new!

So, first, I took the immensely empowering step of throwing out all that JUNK. The late-night infomercial business definitely took a hit that day. Out with the old way, and in with the new!

With that simple action, I reclaimed the driver's seat in my health and wellness journey. I knew at that moment I would find success on my own terms, not relying on gimmicks or gadgets. I would be traveling a different road than I had ever traveled before. It was frightening, yes—but I was ready for the challenge.

Key to my journey was the overall drive to understand and experience the power of my brain and my body, and I knew this required a shift in my mindset. I call it the YES! Mindset, and it required that I create a new relationship with food, with fitness, and with me and my beliefs. I had to take a moment to truly know and appreciate *myself.*

To get out of the negative thought-loop nightmare and create a lasting transformation, I embarked on the task of identifying my true desires. I discovered I no longer desired the love and acceptance of others based upon my weight, but rather *I desired the love and acceptance of myself,* regardless of my size.

This decision eventually led me to become a fitness coach and trainer so I could help others get off their own Yo-Yo paths. Years later, I now help clients truly feel their bodies and experience the wonder of their muscles.

For those of us who rarely allow themselves to slow down, take in their environment, and just feel everything the body is experiencing, please know that these things are key to advancing your wellness journey.

This simple method unlocked the vision for what was possible for me and, later, what was possible for all my clients. There

> God had a unique plan for me, and now I was ready to step into it. I could use my own darkness to bring others into their light.

was hope. I was not destined to continue reliving the negative thought loop tied to the Yo-Yo life, nor was I destined to let my pain trap me in living old habits.

God had a unique plan for me, and now I was ready to step into it. I could use my own darkness to bring others into their light.

The YES! System

My YES! System is not a diet.

I repeat—**it is not a diet!** The YES! System is a lifestyle. It is simple yet powerful: "Commit. Do. Live."

1. **Commit to your true self** and develop that YES! Mindset. I will show you how to do that in this book.

Committing includes getting to know your authentic self and facing your pain. To know your pain's origins is to take a giant step toward creating a life where nothing can stand in your way.

> To know your pain's origins is to take a giant step toward creating a life where nothing can stand in your way.

2. **Do the work.** This work will include developing and growing your positive YES! Mindset through several practices I will teach you, which will allow you to experience that ultimate brain-body connection.

3. **Live your new, authentic life.** For years, I have led my clients on paths that incorporate life-altering habits, nourishing the mind and the body.

By embracing the power of YES! I said "Yes" to a new YES! Mindset, a new YES! Body, and a new YES! Lifestyle. I threw out all the trappings of my prior Yo-Yo existence and committed myself to a new process that revealed new possibilities and a vibrant vision of the future. I got to know my body and its capabilities and to understand my brain and its role in securing sustained changes. As a result, I am now free from any physical and emotional limitations that society places on aging. I am free to live my passions. There is nothing I can't do.

Now, what brings me the greatest joy is being able to share the YES! System and its life-changing techniques with you. You can change your life, too. You can be free to live your own passions.

The only question is:

Are you ready?

> **The YES! Take-Away:** *Shine the light on your pain so it can no longer keep you in the dark.*

THE 'YO YO' LIFE

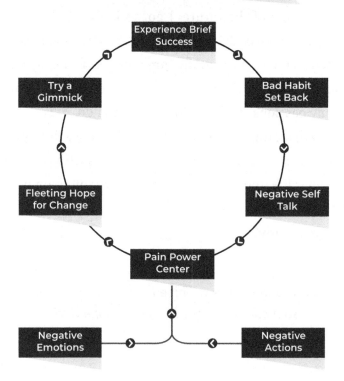

CHAPTER 2

CHOOSE HOPE—OWN YOUR CHOICES

*Attitude is a choice. Happiness is a choice. Optimism is a
choice. Kindness is a choice. Giving is a choice. Respect is a
choice. Whatever choice you make makes you. Choose wisely.*
—ROY T. BENNET, *THE LIGHT IN THE HEART*

Choose Hope

What does hope look like? Hope is defined by *Merriam-Webster's
Dictionary* as "desire accompanied by expectation of or belief
in fulfillment."[4] By making choices that break old habits and
create new norms, our hope edges ever closer to becoming our
reality. The road to finding hope is through the choices we make.
Choices open the window of opportunity. When the choices you
make close that window, you end the possibility of change and
enter a world of false living and limited thinking.

---

4   Merriam-Webster, s.v. "Hope," accessed March 17, 2021, https://www.merriam-
     webster.com/dictionary/hope.

> It is with hope and a positive outlook that possibilities are unleashed, and desires become clear.

It is with hope and a positive outlook that possibilities are unleashed, and desires become clear.

But watch out! Hope can be challenged by old, familiar routines and troublesome habits. If you walk in the unconscious state—the state whereby you don't "live life" but instead "let life live you," old habits can limit your thinking and send you back down the rabbit hole to the land of comfort and continued failure.

Limiting thinking kills hope.

Our Choices—The Hard Truth

One of the hardest things we can do is accept our own roles in the lives we've built. This is especially true when we are not particularly proud of certain aspects of our lives. But through our choices, whether we are proud of them or not, we write the words, the sentences, and the paragraphs that fill our life's chapters with either conscious effort or mindless actions.

Every time I decided to cheat on an eating plan, that was a choice. Every time I quit an exercise program or routine, that was a choice. Every time I did not follow what I had committed to doing, that was a choice.

Every time you put something in your mouth that hurts your body in the long run that is a choice. With each choice comes the sting of disappointment and frustration, along with a cascade of emotions and thoughts, both rational and irrational. "Why can't I just do it?" you ask. "Why me?"

Almost every client I have worked with laments the reasons why they have failed in the past.

Many people live an *unconscious existence* related to their health. They rely on old habits (*emotional, physical, and mental*), norms, and routines to guide their choices—which means they keep making the same old choices.

When your routines don't serve you, it can feel at times like you're running on a hamster wheel—working so hard and getting nowhere.

When I held a fitness class at RWJ Beth Israel Medical Center, many members expressed that they felt that "hamster-wheel" feeling. As doctors, nurses, and hospital staff, their crazy work schedules often led them to skip meals, make unhealthy food choices, have poor posture, breathe inadequately, and skip exercise. Many of them, while so dedicated to patient care, had the habit of forgoing self-care and thus neglecting their long-term health.

The common question was: How can I fit my self-care into this crazy schedule? My answer was and is: How can you not?

Often, routines don't serve you precisely because they are unchallenging. My training client, Ellie, did the same exercise repeatedly. It neither challenged her body nor her mind, and she saw no results. That led her to mistakenly believe that body change was impossible—yet it was only impossible because she was doing the same routine over and over.

Good Choices + Hope = Endless Possibilities
Regardless of the challenge we all face, the one constant is hope.

Hope represents the possibility to do better. Hope enables the reality of endless growth and change and the achievement of overall balance within our lives. The truth is that the choices we make today represent the changes we bring forth tomorrow. If your choices are not bringing you different results, you have to examine their origin. If you keep making the same basic choices to do variations of the same routines, your choices need to change.

Own Your Choices

How do you find hope in the midst of bad, ill-advised choices? The good news is that the choices we make don't have to be negative—but we need to be aware of the choices we're making and their results.

At one point, I had to make the tough decision to leave my singing career due to the vocal challenges I was experiencing. This was after I had left a thirteen-year career as a state and federal prosecutor—and as you might imagine, the concept of changing careers again weighed heavily upon me. I was just at the beginning of my singing career and had developed such a love of jazz, Broadway, and opera.

I felt as though my voice had betrayed me, but I had to accept the role I played in that result. I knew I had not taken as good care of my vocal cords as I should have during those brief magical performances, and that misuse led to the difficulties I experienced.

My training clients have also had to accept similar responsibility for their own choices. Tai, a participant in my RWJ Beth

Israel group, originally felt that the stress of school, work, and family were the reason for her lack of fitness. At the time, she was working full-time at RWJ Beth Israel and attending school for an advanced degree while being a wife and a mom of school-aged children. Her plate was full.

Tai's YES! Mindset breakthrough came through her realization that she wasn't giving herself "me time." Self-care had taken a back seat to all other responsibilities, and without that time commitment, personal fitness was an unattainable goal. Tai's breakthrough was her realization that her decision not to schedule fitness was a choice. The choice of not prioritizing personal wellness and health was on her. It was no one's fault but Tai's.

The good news is that by taking ownership of her choices, Tai also took ownership of her fitness. In consistently working out three to four times a week, she gained muscle mass, increased her balance and energy levels, and over a six-month period, lost over twenty pounds. In the process, Tai gained a deeper understanding of self—the positive attributes that make up her Inner Core. Tai became a Relentless Warrior in her battle to become healthy.

Similarly, when Delores became a participant in my senior health class, she also learned how to claim her Relentless Warrior status. She entered my program needing to learn how to eat and to move in ways that would advance her health. Delores's doctor had told her that she was obese and pre-diabetic, and that diagnosis scared her.

Since childhood, Delores was accustomed to eating a hearty, carb-filled breakfast, lunch, and dinner, followed by a healthy dose of dessert. Bad habits began young and continued into adulthood. Once in my program, Delores committed to adopting healthy habits, limiting her sweets, reading and understanding nutrition labels, setting goals, and exercising three to five times per week. Through her commitment and consistent work in my group each week, within seven months, Delores became thirty pounds lighter and is no longer pre-diabetic.

According to Delores, she is happy, healthy, and confident in her ability to set and reach goals. Her favorite saying is, "Fitness has no age attached to it—there's no age limit to a fit mind or a fit body."

That's a YES! Journey!

What if we were all super-focused on advancing habits that would launch us towards our goals? What if, before every choice we make, we ask:

1. *Does this choice unleash personal possibilities?*
2. *Does this choice bring positivity into my life?*
3. *Does this choice align with who I am?*

The simple act of asking these questions can help you not to make choices you may later regret. By asking these questions, you will begin to accept the consequences your choice may bring.

After making a bad decision, did you ever just say, "**This is all on me, and I take full responsibility for my choice**"? It is not the fault of another person, a difficult situation, a place, or a thing. After all, it is so much easier to blame anything other than ourselves.

How many of us have blamed our bad behavior on family, spouse, work, or "forces beyond my control"?

Taking ownership of your choices can be both empowering and fearful simultaneously. "I" ate the cake. "I" stopped going to the gym. "I" own the extra pounds, the muscle loss, the lack of self-awareness. Though difficult and challenging, full self-acceptance is equally liberating, and it is a necessary first step toward hope and change.

What do you take ownership of?
We all hope to be as healthy as we can be, inside and out. Every client I have trained has desired to stress less, to sleep soundly, to move more, to eat healthily—all crucial desires to maintain overall health. Whether it was one of my senior wellness groups, individual clients, or the variety of church groups for whom I have created fitness classes and programs, everyone wanted to find balance: a way to age with health, grace, and freedom. One of the dreams many of my program participants have expressed most is their desire for the freedom to do things for themselves while serving others.

In the opening credits of the old "Jetsons" cartoon, George Jetson is seen running with his dog on a treadmill, unable to get it to stop. Like George, you might be asking how you can "get off this crazy thing"?

How can you finally put old habits behind you and just move forward?

Three Unproductive Choice Categories

When faced with a challenge, how do you make your choice? What is your decision-making process?

In general, the choices we make about our health often fall into a few categories. Which describes you?

1. The "Medical Industry" Choice

Of course, having amazing medical care is essential to maintaining good overall health. However, if you rely on the medical industry to solve all your problems rather than personally committing to your health, this choice category may not be serving you well. Typically, if this is your go-to choice style, with every ache and pain, you **"flock to the doc"** for immediate relief. Time to medicate, medicate, medicate. Sedate the body and eliminate all remnants of pain. While that can provide some relief, it will never address the complete solution. Masking pain simply shields the reality of what the body truly needs, and that shield is only temporary.

2. The "Go with the Flow" Choice

This choice basically amounts to living a life of a zombie—existing but not truly living. Have you ever had a zombie moment? Maybe you don't remember what you did the day before or how you got from one location to another. Zombies live unconscious lives, unaware of the beauty around them.

This existence-only life aimlessly follows societal norms and trends. So, if the norms tell you aging brings creaky bones, worn-out joints, low energy, and a retirement mentality, you go with the flow. When you live to exist, you accept society's plan, whether it serves you or not.

To break this pattern is to be in tune with your true inner self.

3. The "Negative Thought Loop" Choice

The final choice represents those who internalize their own negative beliefs and thoughts, creating a negative thought loop. This negative internal dialogue can take over your entire existence, becoming draining and emotionally destructive. After all, with this choice, "no" becomes prominent in your language, and you will find yourself saying "No, I can't," "No, I won't," "No, I shouldn't," and "Not for me" more often than not. The internalized "no" represents the loss of hope.

Own Your Choices (Exercise)

1. What choice type do you live in regarding your health? (List all that apply.)

   _____

   _____

   _____

   _____

   _____

   _____

   _____

2. Now think about two or three specific results making those negative choices have brought. For each result, identify two positive alternative choices you could make instead in similar future situations.

_____

_____

_____

_____

_____

3. What decisions regarding your health habits do you want to take ownership of now?

_____

_____

_____

4. What positive choice—an action you are ready to take (physical, emotional, mental)—will you claim **right now**?

Physical _____

Emotional _____

Mental _____

Ownership = Empowerment

It is time to own your choices. Accepting ownership is your pathway to reclaiming your power. There is true power when we accept the decisions we make. It is not a question of fault or blame, nor is it a moment of giving all the reasons for our poor choices. Accepting ownership means that in spite of issues of fault or good reason for bad choices, it was *your decision*. It was *your choice*, and any fallout from that choice belongs to you.

That's power!

Now, think about this: *What if you could change "no" to "yes"?*

The choices we make are the gateway to the actions we take, and those actions create the reality we live in. The good news is that no matter our previous choice—or our feelings of regret, frustration, disappointment, and self-doubt—there is always hope in our ability to change and grow. That hope can serve as the launch pad to positive transformational change.

Find the Possible; Reject the Obstacle

Negative Excuses

Part of being aware of our choices is being aware of the choices we make, even in the ways we think. Our limiting thoughts often disguise themselves as practical-sounding excuses that, if allowed, will stand in the way of change.

Below are some examples of these kinds of excuses.

"It's a Gimmick."

One thing I always ask is whether an offer is some fly-by-night, quick-fix gimmick. That's not always a bad question. That concern was exactly what led me to throw so many false promises (in the form of useless junk) into the trash. Those products represented empty claims designed to tap into the compelling emotional need not to fail again. Many were late-night infomercial fly traps created to capture the vulnerable, and I once was one of the vulnerable.

I, therefore, understand why anyone would ask that question, and I am dedicated to not producing those false hopes.

First, think about what a gimmick really is. Most gimmicks rely on being quick fixes. As you remember, I don't promise a quick fix—because I personally know they don't work. Instead, I asked you in Chapter 1 to commit, do the work, and live the lifestyle. You don't get real change without earning it, as much as we all wish otherwise.

"I Don't Have Time."

The idea of not having enough time is perhaps the most common excuse used to prevent positive change.

"I don't have time to exercise." "I don't have time to eat healthily." "I don't have time to add one more thing to my busy schedule." I've heard all of these, and more.

We give time to the things we deem important. When my clients tell me their time challenges, I ask:

What price is your health worth?

What are you willing to do to experience more energy?

What are you willing to do to sleep better—to eat healthily and stress less?

"I can't do it." "I don't know where to start." This negative mindset has you quitting even before you begin. "I can't" acts as a false protector against the possible pain of failure. After all, you can't fail if you never try. But, if you never try, you can never succeed. It is time to commit to your success.

> *"The most important thing in life is to stop saying,*
> *'I wish,' and start saying, 'I will.' Consider nothing*
> *impossible, then treat possibilities as probabilities."*
> —CHARLES DICKENS

The Brain-Body Connection

In my role as the Fitness/Wellness Research Coordinator at the Rutgers Aging & Brain Health Alliance (ABHA), I focused on all the elements that lead to ultimate health, which stemmed from the brain to the body, and I will show how it will work for you.

There is a connection between your brain and your body that can help make the seemingly impossible possible. In most people, however, that connection remains untapped. You can harness the information gathered by both your brain and your body about every activity, event, opportunity, and life challenge and use it to move you past obstacles in your decision-making.

This is the type of connection that changes possibilities into probabilities.

As I mentioned earlier, one of the opportunities that I absolutely loved was providing fitness instruction to the medical staff at RWJ Beth Israel Medical Center. Due to the crazy staff schedules, I had to provide quick yet effective, workouts.

Many of the hospital staff worked long hours with limited breaks and had unending stress. They had a million and one reasons why they couldn't work out, and they had schedules that supported those reasons. But my RWJ staff also had a desire to live healthier lives and the willingness to learn how. A willing heart can be a source of great power.

For them, I created, in part, "Five Minutes of Fitness Fun" and "Breathe Fit" (focused body movements through deep diaphragmatic breaths). Every fun exercise routine was designed to reinforce the importance for each participant to feel the connection between their body movements and each muscle they used. As they felt each exercise, they began to understand the brain-body connection.

The brain-body connection enhances your brain's ability to direct energy to move your body and to respond to its ever-changing demands.

You can't move without the brain. Comatose people can't move because their brain function is disconnected from their bodies. The brain-body connection is a process. The pre-motor cortex handles the planning; action then happens through the motor cortex. The muscles activate in the proper sequence and to the correct degree. Coordination is key, and anything that prevents that coordination prevents brain-body freedom.

Every decision you make requires coordination of the whole body to execute that decision. Understanding the process gives you a foothold in understanding your power. When this process is not working properly, your brain says "go," but your body says "no." The result of the YES! System is that when your brain says "go," your body says YES!!! We take your emotional desire to do something and turn it into physical and emotional action.

Exercise Your Power

To get a sense of your power, try this simple exercise: Set your timer for four minutes, put on some upbeat music, and prepare to move your body. Since cardio-based exercises are not only heart-healthy but also have been shown to foster brain health, try to increase your heart rate while alternating between:

- One minute of high-knee marching in place *(or running in place if you are ready for that added challenge)*.

- One minute of jumping jacks *(or jumping rope if you are ready for that added challenge)*.

- Repeat the sequence while steadily increasing your pace. While doing the exercise, repeat the words "Yes, I can!" and focus on the benefits you are bringing to both your brain and body. You will be amazed at how challenging four minutes of exercise with focused intensity can be.

Once complete, take time to acknowledge what you have accomplished. Doing this simple exercise was a choice—a positive choice, and your body will thank you for it. The more you mentally reward yourself for the positive choices you make, the more power you will have to reject the negative.

Science Speaks

Exercise can boost the brain and the body. Physical activity can enhance cognition. The brain and body work together as a machine, one designed to move through space efficiently, walking, moving, and maintaining balance. It can also lower the risk of the adverse effects of aging.[5]

When you follow the steps, your life will transform. It has transformed me, it has transformed my clients, and it can transform you.

As Barbara Kingsolver said in *Animal Dreams*, "The very least you can do in your life is figure out what you hope for. And the most you can do is live inside that hope…"

It is time to live inside your hope!

> **The YES! Take-Away:** *Own Your Choices, or Your Choices will Own You.*

---

5   Louis Bherer, Kirk I. Erickson, and Teresa Liu-Ambrose. "A Review of the Effects of Physical Activity and Exercise on Cognitive and Brain Functions in Older Adults." *Journal of Aging Research* 2013 (2013): 1-5.

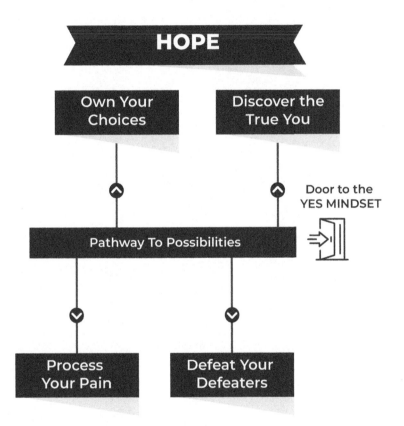

CHAPTER 3

ENTER THE POSITIVITY ZONE—
THE YES! MINDSET

"Life begins at the end of your comfort zone."
—NEALE DONALD WALSCH

Turn Negative to Positive

Living in our hope gives us the strength to confront the negative internal voices and thoughts that lie within each of us. The key is to learn how to turn the negative into the positive. "I can't" transforms to "I can." "I won't" transforms to "I will," and "no" becomes "yes." By replacing each negative with three to five positive thoughts, you begin to create an environment conducive to positive living, and you move towards achieving a YES! Mindset.

But remember: Whether you are aware or not, negative voices play in times of stress and mental challenge. The ones that play loudest are those that have *not been identified*, for they have the greatest power. Unlike the excuses we looked at in the previous chapter, these relate to hidden fears or assumptions, usually coming from your previous pain.

My client Ellie is a great example of someone who has worked hard to transform limiting thoughts. Having suffered a painful and near-crippling back injury years before, she lived in constant fear of re-injuring her back. For years, she allowed these powerful negative voices to limit her fitness endeavors to include only exercises she felt were "safe." Even the thought of adding new fitness movements often made her feel anxious, which then caused more tension in her body. Her fear created a cycle of limitation and more fear that frustrated her and prevented her from fully enjoying family activities. Walking a long distance was out of the question.

My work with Ellie focused on transforming her "no" thinking to "YES!" For her body, we incorporated exercises with fitness bands to increase strength and reinforce proper movements and alignment. But we also worked on freeing her mind from limiting thoughts and replacing them with the possibilities of growth and change. She worked on envisioning herself as the athlete she had the potential to be.

Not only does Ellie now take regular long walks, but she and her husband also went on a five-hour hike. Coming from back pain that had on occasion sidelined her for weeks, this was a great triumph.

"I do more now than I ever did before," Ellie told me. "I claim that 'Superwoman' title... I know I can do it."

What are your limiting thoughts or fears? What opportunities toward advancing your health, career, and relationships

have they caused you to miss? **What power do they have over** *you?* Now is the time to honor yourself by taking the necessary action to eliminate and/or reduce the power that "No" has had over you.

Every time you confront your inner defeaters, you take more of your control back. As your internal strength grows, your YES! Mindset will flourish.

What Stands in Your Way?

Changing the way we think can be a challenge, especially when that change requires that we confront our old way of doing, thinking, and speaking. What can be even more difficult is accepting the reality that those old thoughts and actions stand as the chief obstacles to our ability to grow. There are so many events in our lives where we allow something to prevent us from taking the next steps forward.

To ask for a promotion, to go for a new job, to tell someone you care about them, to step into a difficult challenge – you want to do these things, or you know you should do these things, but something stops you. Whatever the circumstance, it is so important to understand your "what" and your "why." What internal voice blocks your next steps, and why are you allowing yourself to succumb to it?

From Pain Fear to Pain-Free

For some people, as with Ellie, it is fear that stands in the way of real growth and change. Whether it is fear of aches, pains, and injuries that hampers your full-body movement, or fear of failure that hampers your stepping into a new opportunity, if something stands between you and your success, you have to confront it. While the YES! System is not a magic pill against fear, it gives you the tools to address it and create your own YES! Journey.

Unlike those TV ads for copper-infused knee braces with magnets that boast the false promise to magically make your knee pain vanish, your simple commitment to confront your inner thought defeaters, along with your willingness to develop the proper fitness techniques to address your pain, will move you ever closer to attaining your goals and living the life that you desire.

Freedom awaits you, whether it's the freedom to play with your children and grandchildren, go for a walk or a run, or take a fitness challenge. The very thing you fear is the thing that will heal you.

Remember this: **movement is healing,** and **motion is lotion.**

If you're waiting for your pain to magically go away before you get on the path to health and full physical function, you will spend a lifetime waiting. To get over your fear, no matter how it tries to stop you, you just need to act.

If you are willing to learn how your brain can assist in changing your body, and make the commitment to do the work, success can be yours. With a proper fueling plan, the right exercise, and good awareness of your fitness and emotional state, you can make great gains in your overall health.

Science Speaks

The CALM Trial, which stands for Counseling Advice for Lifestyle Management, was a twelve-month study conducted at Stanford University designed to evaluate "how sequential vs. simultaneous diet plans plus PA [physical activity] interventions affected behavior changes."

One group focused on dieting for the first four months, followed by eight months of nutrition and exercise counseling.

Another group received exercise for the first four months, followed by eight months of nutrition and exercise counseling.

Another group received 12 months of nutrition and exercise counseling, and the remaining group received only stress-reduction counseling.

At the end of the study, the only group to meet all goals was the group that focused simultaneously on nutrition and exercise for the entire twelve months.[6]

6   Abby C. King, Cynthia M. Castro, Matthew P. Buman, Eric B. Hekler, Guido G. Urizar, and David K. Ahn. "Behavioral Impacts of Sequentially versus Simultaneously Delivered Dietary Plus Physical Activity Interventions: The CALM Trial." *Annals of Behavioral Medicine* 46, no. 2 (October 2013): 166. https://doi.org/10.1007/s12160-013-9501-y.

Use Pain Against Pain

Sometimes certain kinds of pain can be motivators. My client Cappy sought to improve his physical conditioning so he could escape his physical pain. However, he was motivated by the mental pain he was feeling at the thought of not being able to take care of and actively play with his grandchildren due to his physical state.

I designed a program for Cappy that shattered his self-limiting thoughts about aging and provided a daily routine focusing on Healthy Healing Habits (the "H2H"). This included exercises using resistance bands, along with a healthy eating schedule.

In addition to developing the YES! Mindset, Cappy focused on improving his posture, building his internal strength, and reimagining the aging process. Not only was he able to be more present for his grandchildren, but he also demonstrated, through his commitment to consistent work, that motion truly is lotion.

Seek Out Your Hidden Pain

Sometimes you get stuck holding onto something painful that someone said or did in the past, or decisions you wish you could undo. To truly move past that pain—to process it—the YES! System requires you to step up and do the following:

1. **Shine a light** on your pain that comes from that event, word, or thought so you could take away the hidden power that pain may hold.
2. **Identify** then separate the emotion attached to that pain and write it down.

3. **Recognize** the positive lessons learned from the pain and live in the positive emotions attached to those lessons.

4. **Allow** the positive emotions to replace any negatives feeling that once had power over you.

For me, my "MACK" experience, along with other issues of bullying in my youth, really affected me deeply. Even though I did not walk around focusing on my past, without realizing it, my past was focused on limiting my health and my dreams.

The YES! System essentially re-trains your brain so you can revisit that pain in a new way and in the end, transform it to something positive. You will remove the pain's power source against you and make it work for you. As Joel Osteen said, "You may have had unfair things happen to you, but the depth of your pain is an indication of the height of your future."

Be Consistent to See Results

Consistency is key. For some, the challenge of remaining focused on our health and wellness path can seem insurmountable. But let me tell you a secret—the key is not willpower. Willpower does not work, but accountability does. When you think about accountability, you might envision a fitness trainer or coach. Being accountable to another person can be extremely helpful. However, nothing can compare to finding accountability from within.

Internal Accountability Is Vital

Internal accountability is an essential element of the YES! Mindset. Willpower is a desire, even a decision, to do something. However, you make progress by actually doing, not by wishing to do. If you don't hold yourself accountable, willpower means nothing.

"Willpower as an independent cause of behavior is a myth," according to Dr. Michael R. Lowe, a professor of clinical psychology at the MCP Hahnemann University in Philadelphia. It is a behavior approach and a positive approach to change that is most important.[7]

Internal accountability requires taking a deep dive into what makes you you, and then strengthening your areas of weakness and supporting your areas of strength. Become accountable to your authentic self, and you will realize when you are letting that self down. The connection between your brain and your body is your inner power source to sense your authentic self, hear when you are not true to it, and perform in ways that uphold it.

Internal accountability, once adopted, can last a lifetime. The YES! Mindset takes you down the path to discover this internal power source and use it to cement lifelong change.

The Negative Voices Within

As one of the keys to achieving the YES! Mindset, you have to be willing to confront your inner negative voices. Otherwise, these can trap you in an almost endless maze of internal twists and turns that never lead to what you truly desire. Negative voices and thoughts can convince you that you are not good enough—not

---

7   Jane Fritsch, "Scientists Unmask Diet Myth: Willpower." *The New York Times*, October 5, 1999. https://www.nytimes.com/1999/10/05/health/scientists-unmask-diet-myth-willpower.html

good enough for that job or opportunity, for that relationship, or to meet your fitness and health goals.

Seven Steps for Transforming Negative Voices

Transforming negative voices is easier than you might think. Just do the following:

1. **Acknowledge** that the voice or thought is there.
2. **Listen** to what it is telling you.
3. **Dissect** the inconsistencies and false arguments.
4. **Accept** the truisms.
5. **Find** forgiveness.
6. **Learn** and grow.
7. **Flip** the Script—replace negative with positive.

> These steps help place you in the driver's seat of your mind, giving you back your power over your future.

These steps help place you in the driver's seat of your mind, giving you back your power over your future.

Acknowledge It

One day when I was a federal prosecutor, ten defense attorneys and I were in court arguing a legal matter when the presiding judge announced he would keep us in court late into the evening until the matter was resolved. I became panicked. My two-year-old son's daycare, located just across the street, would close in ten minutes, and I would be late in picking him up.

I privately informed the judge of my dilemma, and he allowed me to go—but I was still twenty minutes late. My negative internal voices and corresponding emotions took hold over me. I heard, "You are such a bad mom. You are always late. You will never be as good a mom as your mother. Your mother would never have left you like this…" And you can imagine how I felt, with that internal dialogue going on.

In situations like this, it can be easy to just try to focus on solving the problem and ignore the voice. But that won't work. Instead, you must realize you have these negative voices that can play in your subconscious mind, influencing behavior and preventing you from successfully completing your goals. Without recognizing the negative voice, you unwittingly give it power over you in ways you cannot even contemplate. You become a marionette on strings being moved and controlled by forces you are unaware of. The first step to breaking those strings is to acknowledge the power with which the negative voice has operated in your life—as in the story of Pinocchio, breaking the strings creates a new reality.

Listen to It

In your new state of truth through acknowledgement and awareness, you must now listen to that negative voice without interruption and without emotion. Our normal reaction is to try to quiet the voice immediately or drown it with unhealthy food, drink, or some other negative behavior. We are often even inclined to respond by agreeing with it and tacking on additional negative thoughts, taking ourselves to an even deeper spiral of emotions. Don't let that happen. Just listen and learn. To lessen the power of that negative tune, you must listen to the complete thought and not let emotion move you.

After all, the reason that thought comes up often is because it has power. Until you let it play out fully, you will never understand the full power it has. Listen, and get ready to reclaim your power.

Dissect It

Once that negative voice is able to run its full course, you will become aware of **three different parts of its message**:

- Inconsistencies,
- Lies, and
- Truisms.

After listening fully, you will be surprised at the ridiculous claims those thoughts contain. Where you hear "never" or "always," you will be sure to find inconsistencies.

In pursuing my cases while both a state and federal prosecutor, I had to find the truth and discern when someone or something was full of inconsistencies and lies. The situation with my inner thoughts was no different.

When you listen without emotion, *you become the prosecutor* of your negative voices and learn to identify their inconsistencies and outright lies. With each inconsistency, that negative voice loses credibility. With every lie, that negative voice loses reliability. As their credibility diminishes, so does their power.

In my situation, I confronted the lies and inconsistencies. I was not a "bad mom," nor was I "always" late. Those were blatant lies that could be refuted by multiple counter examples.

However, the negative thoughts could not have gained such power or for some, operated over countless years if the truth were not embedded within the lies.

What is the truth embedded in your negative thought(s)?

In my case, I wasn't *always* late, but I *was* late a lot. That was true. And my being late did cause distress, not only to my son but also to the staff at the daycare. That was the reality.

Accept the Truth

Until I faced the truth and forgave myself for the mistakes I made, I was stuck in the negative thought loop that could appear at any moment of personal or situational weakness.

> When you accept the truth that underpins the lies, your acceptance creates a magical moment of possible transformation and growth.

When you accept the truth that underpins the lies, your acceptance creates a magical moment of possible transformation and growth.

Now that you've accepted the truism without the other false thoughts, you've stripped the negative thought of its power. The truth may be a "tough pill to swallow," but doing so is essential to moving forward.

Acceptance of that truth empowers you to figure out solutions to meet the challenge. If it is a career-oriented negative thought, maybe the truth is that you need additional training or certification or degree. If you are chronically tardy, maybe the solution is to find a better support system that will help you in the areas where you are deficient.

Forgive

My faith requires forgiveness—not only forgiveness of others, but also forgiveness of myself. And that last part became crucial to getting past the negative internal dialogue.

Although I had so many counter-examples showing that I was not a bad mom, those did not refute the fact that I was frequently late to the daycare. By accepting my truth and forgiving myself for not always doing as I hoped I would, I lessened both the sting and power of that thought. I broke the loop that my negative internal voice operated within. **No more auto-play**!

To all those busy parents taking on multiple responsibilities, take time to forgive yourself and **power up** on all that is positive in your life.

Learn and Grow

If we do this thing called life correctly, we will be students, open to learning the rest of our lives. It is work to confront our own negative voices, and to change them from negative to positive requires commitment and dedication to the YES! System.

Even though our inner voice may sometimes falsely accuse us, as mentioned earlier, it may also bring forth truth. When we have fallen short as a parent, a child, a friend, an employee, or as a human being, our failing can be difficult to face. However, facing that difficulty brings forth possibilities for growth and change.

Maybe it opens the door to more education, a training program, counseling, or perhaps a new opportunity or relationship not previously envisioned. The key is to make the necessary changes that move us forward in our personal journeys. What began as a negative has the opportunity to spur positive, exciting change.

Flip the Script

Flipping the script has two meanings. First, when you think back on that negative thought, remember the strength you brought forth to move through that experience. Focus on the power of your character you had to ignite to move forward as you traversed that difficult moment.

When you think about your inner power, how does that make you feel? Make note of that feeling so next time, if and when your mind wanders to a negative thought, you will focus on that positive feeling.

Second, flipping the script allows you to see each new situation in a positive light. You take what you would have thought of as bad and flip it to good. Take what was a bad habit and adopt a good one. "I can't" becomes "I can," and "I won't" becomes "I will."

When my client Marcella joined my senior health program, she was struggling with a recent weight gain due in part to physical inactivity and poor food choices. She felt stalled in her health journey, stuck in this new weight, and frustrated that she had let it happen.

Whereas Marcella spent much of her early adulthood maintaining a healthy weight, she had recently fallen into bad habits of limited exercise and overeating, and those habits were taking a toll on her health. She became extremely self-conscious, camouflaging those extra pounds around her waistline with bulky jackets and sweaters.

But Marcella couldn't camouflage her issues from herself, and her attempt to hide only gave those negative thoughts more power over her. This is why camouflage never works.

She finally realized she had lost sight of the importance of her health, and she wanted to get her healthy body back. She was ready for change. She was ready to flip her script.

Marcella adopted the YES! Mindset. This mindset helped her to own her choices, both good and bad, and to focus on her goals. With that ownership, she could no longer try to hide her choices or blame her weight gain on friends, work stress, or other life situations. The fault was hers, and hers alone, and that acceptance served as her pathway to personal strength and empowerment. She used the tools of the program to celebrate the components of her Inner Core and find her internal motivation and focus.

Marcella changed her relationship with eating/fueling and exercising. That change, along with her renewed focus, enabled her to lose twelve pounds in two-and-a-half months.

Once the negative inner script is shut down, the peace that follows will allow those voices to work in harmony with, rather than in conflict with you. That negative internal dialogue created ongoing conflict between your body and your brain, leading to feelings of fear, doubt, sadness, and worry.

Using the YES! System helps to shut down that negative inner script that reflected the constant conflict between the brain and the body. Shut it down and diminish the power it once held over you. The harmony that can thrive once the conflict is resolved allows the body to de-stress, reset, and experience inner peace. Lasting inner peace occurs once your Inner Core, thoughts, beliefs, character, and chosen actions are balanced and aligned with each other.

Identify Your Inner Defeaters

To move forward on your YES! Journey, ask yourself:

1. What are your inner defeaters? What do your negative voices say to you?

_____

_____

_____

_____

_____

_____

2. What opportunities for personal growth has this process revealed to you?

   a. _____

   _____

b. _____

_____

c. _____

_____

The YES! Take-Away: Process your pain, defeat your inner defeater, and find the positive in what was negative. When you know who you are, you can ignite the power within.

CHAPTER 4

WHO ARE YOU?
WHAT IS YOUR TRUE DESIRE?

"Nothing can dim the light which shines from within."
—MAYA ANGELOU

Your Road Forward

Now that you have committed to your YES! Mindset and are on this journey, it is important to recognize where you have been and what steps you must take to experience sustained change.

So far:

- You have acknowledged the pain that has served as a barrier to sustained change in your life and have created a new positive relationship with that experience.

- You have stepped into your YES! Journey of hope by identifying your negative choices, and you have committed your future to making better, more positive choices that will unleash your life's possibilities. You have owned your choices and taken responsibility for the results.

- You have begun the process to confront and tackle your inner defeaters—words, thoughts, and experiences that created an environment of limited thinking and limited opportunities.

> The road to self-discovery begins with a simple question: What do you really want?

But before you can fully activate the YES! Mindset, you need to be clear on who you are. What makes you "you"? You must understand and embrace your authentic self and continue the process of finding your inner peace.

The road to self-discovery begins with a simple question: What do you really want?

Your Inner Core

To truly find your inner peace, you must explore your core.

But what does that mean?

The things you want and value most, and the ways in which you express those desires and values, reflect your true self, your Inner Core. That question, "What do you want?" is so simple, yet many find answering it a great challenge. It is amazing how many people never ask themselves that question. By not doing so, they deprive themselves of the opportunity to live their true desires. The quest for personal understanding opens possibilities for incredible growth. To know your true desires requires an understanding of self.

Who are you? What do you stand for, and what defines the essence of you?

I remember the first time I asked myself those questions. I had been a practicing attorney for well over twelve years and had had the opportunity to prosecute a variety of cases and speak on areas of the law. I found it fascinating, yet I had an uneasy feeling that there was more. I did not know how to articulate it, but I was missing something.

Everything crystallized for me one evening at an attorney career mixer. Everyone was introducing themselves as they always had at similar events over the years. They were reciting their names, career titles, and positions, as well as the companies, organizations, and firms they represented. But this evening, I heard it in a different way. As I listened, I realized that no one was really introducing *who* they were. It was just names, titles, and positions, and we would all leave that space not knowing anyone's true self.

At that moment, I became committed to discovering, defining, researching, understanding, and living by who I truly am.

So I ask you again: Who are you? Are you your possessions? Your education? Your career? Your rewards? Your family? Your friends? At your core, what matters most?

To fully embrace the YES! Mindset, you must fully embrace yourself. Begin by decluttering your mind and your life of things that do not define or serve you, so you can make way for things that do—including other people.

Stop and determine:

1. Your loves and passions
2. Your talents and gifts
3. Your wants and desires

Never forget what envelops all of these factors.

Character is King

During this time of self-discovery, you must focus on your character and your value system. They matter. How you see the world and your ability to connect and grow hinge greatly on the strength of your character. Be compassionate, and you will find that people will respond in kind. Be empathetic and understanding, and others will also gain in their ability to understand you. You can only ask for what you are willing to give.

What does your character look like, and what are the moral principles that guide your actions?

I remember reading *The Picture of Dorian Gray* by Oscar Wilde. In that book, Dorian's portrait magically reflected the truth of his character, changing over time based on his actions. As he aged, it grew frightful, reflecting every negative thought, ill deed, and deceitful act that was imprinted on his soul.

It is imperative to live your true character and to celebrate and nurture those values that uplift yourself and others. As you ask yourself the tough questions, your vision of yourself will become clearer, and you will learn to live in harmony with those factors that best describe the true you.

This journey into self-understanding is a key process in fortifying your YES! Mindset and moving you towards achieving your desires. You have to know who you are to attain what you want.

All of these components are what make you a unique individual. Your passions, loves, talents, gifts, and desires, along with your character values, all inform and empower you.

For me, this exploration unearthed my passion for singing and acting and cemented my courage to leave the law in pursuit of my dream. It later grounded the inner strength, grit, and determination to enter this wonderful career in the world of health and wellness.

Having the courage to relive your pain, find your hope, challenge your choices, confront your inner defeaters, and journey in self-discovery is the path the YES! Mindset and will give you the necessary internal strength needed to support any direction your life may take.

Live Positively

To maximize this new and rich understanding of yourself, immersing yourself in a positive environment becomes essential. Positive brings positive, so grow your positive YES! Mindset and nourish it with a commitment to the following **four steps:**

1. Think positive thoughts.
2. Speak positive words.
3. Take positive actions.
4. Surround yourself with the most positive people.

When you take these four steps, not only will you advance towards your goals, but also your ability to combat negative people, negative environments, and negative thoughts will grow. You will be on the path of breaking the vortex of negativity and your dependence on prior behavior and old habits.

Science Speaks

According to a behavioral research study, positive ideation reduced the *frequency* of worry-related thoughts, allowing participants to disengage from the negativity of worry, focusing instead on positive content. These findings converge on the idea that repeated practice in replacing worry with positive ideation can counter the intrusive and distressing properties of worry.[8]

Hidden Gem to a Positive Mind

One of the first rules I set with my clients is pivotal to the YES! Mindset, and I now want to set it with you. From this point on, you cannot say anything negative about yourself. That's right! My hidden gem is the rule of no insults, no body-part put-downs, and no negative nicknames. Your life is now an insult-free zone.

8   Claire Eagleson, Sarra Hayes, Andrew Mathews, Gemma Perman, and Colette R. Hirsch. "The Power of Positive Thinking: Pathological Worry Is Reduced by Thought Replacement in Generalized Anxiety Disorder." *Behaviour Research and Therapy* 78 (March 2016): 18. https://doi.org/10.1016/j.brat.2015.12.017

The second part of that is that you must also list five positive adjectives that best describe you and repeat those adjectives daily. If a negative thought rears its ugly head, repeat the five positive adjectives to combat and transform that negative idea.

Be consistent, and it will work. You will choose to focus on what is good in your life when you recognize that focusing on the bad doesn't serve you in the long run. Consistently focusing on positive aspects about yourself will unleash your optimistic mind, moving you from the attitude of the "glass-half-empty" to one of the "glass half-full."

Your Positive Adjectives:

1. _____

2. _____

3. _____

4. _____

5. _____

Body Positive

Positivity expresses itself physically. When the brain and the body thrive on positivity, we feel good, and our posture often reflects our mood. But the reverse is also true. Change your posture, and you change your brain. We are not designed to be bent over, looking down at the ground, breathing shallowly. Being physically positive (with good posture) allows the chest to be upright and open, fostering deep, body-enriching breaths. Your head is kept upright and supported by your kinetic chain of bone, ligament, and postural muscles, and all those body changes also affect your brain, which is able to think more clearly.[9]

Similarly, the positive mindset sends messages to the brain, encouraging the release of endorphins that signal the brain and body to enter a state of joy and relaxation. Tension and stress will dissipate, and a state of homeostasis or brain-body balance will occur. This positivity shepherds in a peaceful nature, and that peace becomes an essential component to experiencing health and wellness.

As I tell all my fitness groups, as the positivity factors set in, you become Kings and Queens of yourself and your environment. You are in charge of yourself. As Royalty, you honor your brain and your body, which is reflected in the way in which you carry yourself. You achieve a poise you did not have before.

Make the Ongoing Commitment

As I already noted in the chapter on choice, to live with a positive outlook is a choice. That choice starts the process of attaining a YES! Mindset, which ultimately leads to that YES! Body. Once you enter the positivity zone, you take a major step towards attaining your true desire. To stay in this zone requires an ongoing commitment. You must:

---

9   Erik Peper, Richard Harvey, Lauren Mason, and I-Mei Lin. "Do Better in Math: How Your Body Posture May Change Stereotype Threat Response." *NeuroRegulation* June 30, 2018 5(2): 72. https://doi.org/10.15540/nr.5.2.67.

1. Live in optimism.
2. Recite your positive adjectives.
3. Be inspirational.
4. Be passionate.
5. Be compassionate.

Now that you know who you truly are, what steps will you take to nourish your Inner Core?

1. Identify three acts of compassion you will perform:

    a. _____

    b. _____

    c. _____

2. List what inspires you.

    _____

    _____

    _____

3. What will you do to be an inspiration to others?

    a. _____

    b. _____

    c. _____

Science Speaks

According to Andrew Newberg, M.D. and Mark Robert Waldman, a single positive or negative word can actually alter your brain. In their book, *Words Can Change Your Brain*, they write:

"If you intensely focus on a word like "peace" or "love," the emotional centers of the brain calm down. The outside world hasn't changed at all, but you will still feel more safe and secure. This is the neurological power of positive thinking, and to date, it has been supported by hundreds of well-designed studies."[10]

The YES! Take-Away: *Know your authentic self and live by your Inner Core.*

---

10   Andrew Newberg, M.D. and Mark Robert Waldman, *Words Can Change Your Brain* (New York, New York: the Penguin Group, 2012), 441.

CHAPTER 5

IT'S TIME TO BREAK OLD HABITS

*"The greatest glory in living lies not in never
failing but in rising every time we fall."*
—NELSON MANDELA

Our behaviors became habits because something made them feel safe and comforting to us. That's why changing them is difficult, even when we admit the habit isn't good. When we form habits that result in things like our being tired, obese, or unfit with high blood pressure and/or diabetes, we may not like the results, but until we shine the light on the reasons why the habits formed, changing them will be an almost insurmountable feat.

Habit Origin

Once you learn your habit's birth point, the reason it formed will be evident. My client Monica's lack of regular workouts sprang from having a job with a challenging work schedule. Being a nurse in management, as well as a wife and mother, posed a daily challenge to carve out health moments dedicated to self-care.

Monica loved ice skating, but with her increased weight and low fitness level, her enjoyment suffered. When she joined my hospital health program, she had back pain, weak core muscles, and limited cardiovascular fitness. She was frustrated and disappointed at how far she had let herself go. It was easy for Monica to choose to care for everyone else over caring for herself. In a way, focusing on others took the attention away from the negative process that was happening to her.

In another example, my client Tai's eating habits were born from over-snacking as a child, and those habits followed her into adulthood, where they served as a comfort to the daily stress common within the hospital environment.

What about you?

As I mentioned before, I had the habit of diet hopping. I was always on the lookout for the latest trend, and this was my habit from the days of the MACK incident. It is what I knew, and I did it without thought or deep contemplation. It had become my safe place. Rather than dealing with any emotions related to my weight, I spent time looking for and trying the latest fad. It was an addiction. I couldn't pass a grocery-store checkout lane without noticing a magazine highlighting some celebrity diet or "fail-safe" method of losing weight.

Sadly, I was comfortable with that routine even though I understood it wasn't serving me.

Three-Day Cabbage Soup Diet, anyone?

We have three types of habits: mental habits, emotional habits, and physical habits. Each impacts the brain and the body. With each type of habit, there are hidden triggers that activate the emotion, thought, or behavior. Not only do we need to discover the habits' origins, but we must also know the type of habit and the triggers that call it to action.

When we understand the habit, we gain the upper hand in taking it from dark to light—from hurtful to helpful. So let's first explore the types of habits and how they manifest.

Mental Habits

Mental habits are often formed in response to situations that we experienced or routines we engaged in consistently over time that we eventually accepted as our "norm." These are internal messages we tell ourselves day in and day out, and they can live within our conscious and subconscious minds.

Our mental habits help us to cope with our environment—situations, people, places, and things—and they can be positive or negative. In their negative form, they can make us physically and mentally sick and crush our dreams, ambitions, and hope for the future.

The good news is that we have the power to turn any negative mental habit positive, but first, we must identify those habits that may be controlling us in an unproductive manner and make an honest assessment of their origins.

Three Common Negative Mental Habits

Do you see yourself in any of these three mental habits?

Mental Habit 1: Perfectionism

Holding oneself (or others) to an impossible standard can create great mental stress. It can also set forth a paradigm of endless perceptions of failure and disappointment. When you find yourself constantly dissatisfied with people who don't measure up or with places and activities that never meet your standards, daily life will be rather unbearable.

> *Mindset Shift:* First, reevaluate your expectations and make sure they are realistic. Then, focus on empathy and compassion for others. It is amazing what you discover when you walk in the shoes of your fellow man. Compassion and understanding of others will set your path for deeper compassion and understanding of yourself. Shift by altering the purpose behind your actions.

Mental Habit 2: Mental Clutter

Unending internal chatter will impede your ability to find clarity and move forward with purpose. When your "thought overload" becomes a paralyzing force, you can feel stuck, unable to move forward in a relationship, career, spirituality, personal growth, or life purpose.

> *Mindset Shift:* It is time to de-clutter and simplify. Focus on those things that are most important in your life, and let go of things that aren't really serving you. Think about the factors in your Inner Core. Now simplify your life so you can live for them. Knowing who you are and owning your Inner Core moves you ever closer to living the YES! Mindset.

Mental Habit 3: Living in Your Head

Living only in your head is a road to endless frustration. You plan to do. You dream of doing. You promise to do. But nothing actually gets done. Without true accomplishments, your life is at a perpetual standstill. That is the same as hamster-wheel living, and if you don't shift your mindset, you will stay stuck.

Mindset Shift: To get out of your head and live the life you were intended to live, not only must you take the steps to discover who you are, as outlined in Chapter 4, but you must also make a daily commitment to be present in your current life rather than in your ideas of it—finding the joy that surrounds you right now. In fact, right now, take a moment to do the Quick Connection Exercise below and see how you feel afterward.

These steps will continually connect you to what is most important in your environment and your relationships and motivate you to live in the present; instead of worrying about the past or being anxious for the future.

Quick Connection Exercise

Here's a great way to connect quickly with your surroundings:

- Take a breath in through your nose and hold for five seconds.

- Exhale through your mouth and hold for five seconds.

- Repeat that process three times.

Emotional Habits

Emotional habits are habits directly triggered by the emotions we experience. Whether it is guilt, failure, boredom, the pursuit of perfectionism, or feelings of regret or loss, our emotional habits are born from those feelings and can become automatic in our lives.

How many of us have felt the sting of failure? When you put all your efforts and time into a project, a job, a relationship or a dream and it fails, what do you turn to for relief? When you are sad, do you try to soothe your mind and body with food or shrink away from doing anything physical? Or is loneliness the feeling that calls upon food for comfort?

When I was a freshman at Tufts University, I had a girl-friend who used food as a comforter. Her transition to college was difficult, and her food of choice was a pint of vanilla ice cream. Fortunately (or unfortunately), we had an ice creamery that delivered into the early morning hours. They sold a lot of ice cream that year.

- What emotion triggers you?
- When you are emotionally triggered, do chips, soda, ice cream, cookies, or other similar foods call your name?

Recognizing and understanding your triggers is key in enabling you to mount a counter-offensive to change habits that hurt into habits that help.

Three Common Emotional Habits

Do you see yourself in any of these three emotional habits?

Emotional Habit 1: Burying and Suppressing Your Feelings

Living a false life by refusing to allow your authentic feelings is a recipe for fake, unfulfilling relationships, lost dreams, lost hope, confusion, stress, and deep personal sadness. It is lonely when you have no true understanding of who you are.

> *Mindset Shift:* The recipe for unearthing your feeling and bringing the truth to the light rests in working on your Pathway to Possibilities, or the P.O.D.D.

- **Process** your pain.
- **Own** your choices.
- **Defeat** your defeaters.
- **Discover** the true, authentic you—God's unique design for your life.

It is part of your road to the YES! System, and you cannot take any shortcuts.

Emotional Habit 2: "Fixing" Unwanted Emotions

Whether you are sad, lonely, angry, frustrated, or experiencing any other unwanted emotion, do you try to nullify it with a quick fix to end that feeling? For some, it is "see food-eat food"—anything that will make them feel better. For others, it could be just the opposite—starving themselves or going on the Banana Diet to feel like they're fixing the problem.

But as we've already seen, there is no food, diet, or product that will comfort you more than superficially nor truly solve your problems. There are no quick fixes. True change takes a commitment to self-work and the willingness to be consistent in your efforts.

Mindset Shift: To shift an unwanted emotion, it is important to know that emotion's origins. Emotions often emanate from pain, and if you don't take ownership of it, those emotions can control you. Remember to process your pain and to shine the light on the emotion so you can follow the steps in Chapter 4 to change that negative emotion into positive power.

Emotional Habit 3: Dwelling in Constant Emotions

When negative emotions run rampant in your brain to the point where they make multiple daily appearances, your body's stress levels can be overwhelming. Not only does stress disrupt sleep, but it can also cause serious health issues such as heart disease, high blood pressure, diabetes, and other illnesses.

Getting lost in the emotional feelings of sadness, anger, regret, disappointment, guilt, or depression can also trigger self-destructive behaviors that bring ongoing, lasting harm to the brain and the body. This stressed, weakened state magnifies your cravings and heightens your need to find emotional relief while diminishing your ability to make good decisions. The good news is that you can change this.

Mindset Shift: By adopting the following three steps, you can begin to gain balance over the negative emotions and eliminate their power over you.

- **Identify your emotional trigger** or triggers and the foods and/or actions that you instantly want to eat/take once that emotion is triggered.

- **Write it down.** Remember—anything you bring out of the darkness and into the light loses power over you.

- **Change the response.** Now that you have identified the trigger, make a conscious choice to replace the usual triggered action with a new action plan that you will do immediately upon the outset of that emotion.

For instance, if sadness triggers you to eat, instead of wandering into the kitchen, as usual, set your new action to take a five-minute walk outside, call a specific friend or family member, or engage in an activity of self-care. Be consistent in enforcing this for yourself, and change will come!

Physical Habits

Physical habits come in many forms. Some physical habits support our health, while others destroy it. It's good to ask yourself how your physical habits are affecting your long-term health. These habits consist of not only things we choose to do but also things we choose not to do.

Common Physical Habits

Do you see yourself in any of these three physical habits?

Physical Habit 1: Laziness or Avoidance

If you rarely move your body unless walking from one room to another, or if you always opt to take the elevator or escalator instead of the stairs, you may be suffering from this habit. Avoiding movement can cause you to lose your physical fitness over the long term. With that loss, you will experience low energy, muscle fatigue, imbalance within the body, and weight gain. Remember, a body at rest stays at rest.

Mindset Shift: Confront laziness or avoidance head-on by adopting a new set of physical habits as your Daily Challenge. This challenge requires you to take the following steps:

- **Spend no more than forty-five consecutive minutes seated.** Get up and walk around to foster ongoing physical activity. That movement will help you avoid stiffness and encourage proper cardiovascular circulation.

- **Take two ten-minute walks each day:** one in the morning and one in the evening. This simple addition to your routine will further your cardiovascular health and aid in proper digestion.

- **Add steps into your day whenever possible.** Park a little further away from the store. Take the stairs instead of the elevator.

Physical Habit 2: "Feast or Famine" Fitness

This happens when your fitness journey consists of starting and stopping fitness routines, fitness classes, gym memberships, personal training, and group training, and it has become a common routine. Sometimes, you are all in—so dedicated and determined! And other times, you do not welcome physical fitness or any type of physical activity as a part of your life.

Is there a way to remain in the feast state and eliminate the famine? The answer is, as you may have guessed, YES! You merely need to reinforce your commitment to move your body.

Mindset Shift: To reverse the "feast or famine" habit, along with applying the other YES! Mindset components, make the following changes:

- **Begin small and build from there.** Big changes often begin with tiny actions. Instead of trying to do everything all at once, reduce the "feast" to a simple "meal." Start with ten minutes of a physical activity that you enjoy. Do that for ten minutes each day, five to seven days each week. After two to four weeks, you should be able to see how that mini-habit can plant the seed for long-term change. Now add another mini-habit.

- **Develop a relationship with your breath.** This relationship will heighten your brain-body connection and help you increase the enjoyment of your chosen physical activities. We'll go into more detail about this in Chapter 7, where you will learn how to breathe deeply, using all chambers of your breath. To strengthen this relationship, commit to five minutes of focused deep breathing daily.

Physical Habit 3: Instant Gratification

Do your impulses drive you into action—or to inaction? Does the need for gratification control your behavior? If you find yourself a slave to your impulses, doing things such as purchasing gimmicks that advertise instant pain relief or going on diet plans that promise overnight weight loss miracles, you already know that they represent false answers. Real, lasting change can only occur when you make a commitment to walk truthfully within your health and wellness journey.

Mindset Shift: Although physical habits are also tied to emotional and mental habits, let's agree to a set of movements and activities that will be done, regardless of whether we want to or not. It sounds backward, but in this case, the doing will lead to the "wanting." The YES! Mindset will elevate and support the "wanting," making the activity something you want to keep doing.

If you are hooked on gimmicks:

- **Avoid infomercials and place yourself on a purchase moratorium.** When I lived the "Yo-Yo life," I loved a gimmick and quick fix promise. My cupboards and closets were at one time full of false promises and lost hopes. They didn't serve me then, and they will not serve you now!

- **Replace your love of the instant with a commitment to forever.** Once you shift into the YES! Mindset, understanding and embracing all that life holds possible for you, you will leave instant impulses behind without a backward glance. You will no longer even listen to them, for they have nothing real to give you.

Reflection Exercise

1. What habits do you need to break? (These may or may not be the common ones listed above.)

Mental: _____

_____

Emotional: _____

_____

Physical: _____

_____

2. What positive mindset shifts are you willing to make?

Mental: _____

_____

Emotional: _____

_____

Physical: _____

_____

The YES! Take-Away: Don't let mental, emotional, or physical habits stand between you and your greatness! Make a mindset shift and replace any bad habits with good ones.

CHAPTER 6

CREATE YOUR YES! VISION

"It is when I struggle that I strengthen. It is when challenged to my core that I learn the depth of who I am."
—STEVE MARABOLI

Your YES! Mindset empowers you to make your own reality. You will be able to transform your goals, dreams, and true desires from the imaginary to the physical—from the dream to reality. You become a Reality Maker, igniting your internal power source. Then you are able to meet all future challenges and confront all future obstacles.

You can achieve this capability simply by performing all of the actions you've committed to thus far to attain your YES! Mindset. The trick is to make those actions your new, ongoing habits. Through the rest of your life, you will continue this positive cycle as you keep processing your pain, owning your choices, defeating your defeaters, and discovering the true you. This work is never finished as you continue to nurture new parts of yourself.

To be a Reality Maker is to have a clear and concise vision for your future. That vision, which is a manifestation of your ideas, your senses, your imagination, and your dreams, will propel you toward your goals. Think of your goals as a trampoline to spring you toward your true desires.

It is time to make your vision clear! It is time to create your own personal YES! Vibrant Vision. Follow the four steps below to solidify your Yes! Vision so that you can state it boldly and with clarity, allowing you then to design the goals that will move you closer to your desires.

Step 1: Heighten Your Senses

In defining your YES! Vision, your ability to tap into each of your senses (sight, sound, touch, taste, smell) is essential. And please note: if any one of these senses is not available to you, the others become even more heightened. Your senses are a gateway toward creating the images tied to your YES! Vision. They provide the textures of taste, sound, smell, and touch, bringing reality to a vision of something that has yet to occur. Essentially, your senses make your YES! Vision feel real right now, and that is powerful.

It is far easier to tap into this power source when you understand and appreciate living in the present. You might ask, "How does living in the present have anything to do with achieving something in the future?" Simple. If you do not know how to enjoy the sights, the sounds, the colors, the textures, and the feeling of things that are right before you—the beauty that lies everywhere you go—then you will never be able to envision your dream in a way to make it real.

Deepening your ability to live in the present will change your life. Each day, we have over 6,200 thoughts that cross our minds —6,200 thoughts![11] If you are not careful, you might spend too many of those thoughts lamenting the past—living in regret-land or imagining ways you could have handled situations better. Or conversely, you might find yourself living in the future, worrying or dreading things that may never come to pass or situations that may never occur.

Either way, all those moments amount to wasted living. They are moments you could have used to advance your dreams, and you can never reclaim them—they are lost forever.

Being present allows you to bask in all the beauty that surrounds you daily. It heightens your ability to truly listen to all that is being said and to feel all that is happening in real-time.

To understand how to be present, do the "Five Minutes of Focus" exercise and begin to let your breath unlock your internal power that will be used to bring clarity to your YES! Vision.

---

11 "Humans Have More than 6,000 Thoughts per Day Psychologists Discover." Newsweek.com, accessed March 20, 2021, https://www.newsweek.com/humans-6000-thoughts-every-day-1517963

Exercise: Five Minutes of Focus

During each day, take five minutes to do the following:

- Stop and take five deep, diaphragmatic breaths.
- Close your eyes and think only of the rich oxygen permeating every cell of your body.
- Open your eyes and take note of all the beauty (the sights, the shapes, the smells, the sounds, the colors) that surrounds you.
- Engage all your senses. Allow your body to feel peace and experience calm.

Afterward, share your experience with at least one other person, or if you are alone, write it down.

What did you experience in your five focused minutes?

_____

_____

_____

Step 2: Use Constructive Daydreaming to Unlock Your YES! Vision

Constructive daydreaming or mind-wandering is an opportunity for your brain to disconnect from a current activity or specific task at hand. It allows your mind to reveal the multiple layers and facets of your dreams. By daydreaming, you help to assure that your vision is not solely the reflection of your daily living or the thought of expectations and limitations others may have placed upon you.

When you constructively daydream, your mind will more fully, beautifully, and freely unearth every aspect of your dream, helping to guarantee that it will have no limits. No more boxes or self-imposed prisons.

According to neuroscience, there is a region in the brain that lights up during daydreaming or mind wandering. Scientists believe this area fosters creative thinking.[12] Allow that creativity to combine with your previously identified loves, passions, and inspirations to help reveal your YES! Vision.

Constructively daydreaming will encourage your brain to release the neurochemicals that foster relaxation and that de-stressed state of being. Great ideas can reveal themselves during a peaceful state. The brain-body connection is always working.

Here is one way this has played out in my life. While an actress, I was thrilled to be cast as Blanche, the title role in the play, *A Streetcar named Desire*, by Tennessee Williams. It was a role I had dreamed about playing since leaving the practice of law to pursue my acting/singing career. It was a role that, early on in an acting class, I was told I could never play due to the color of my skin. Regardless, I had seen myself playing that role long before I was cast.

After getting the part, I was tasked with learning hundreds of pages of text. I remember how my excitement at being selected

12   Sergio Agnoli, Manila Vanucci, Claudia Pelagatti & Giovanni Emanuele Corazza (2018) "Exploring the Link Between Mind Wandering, Mindfulness, and Creativity: A Multidimensional Approach." *Creativity Research Journal*, 30:1: 41-53, DOI: 10.1080/10400419.2018.1411423

dissolved almost immediately into an overwhelming fear that I wasn't up to the task.

To confront this, I used constructive daydreaming to visualize each word and phrase of the play. I also visualized how I would bring the character to life on stage. I used my inspirations from music, dance, ballet, art, and nature. Those images constantly flooded my mind and nourished my soul to capture the true essence of Blanche. I used my character strengths—my tenacity, creativity, and passion—to successfully meet the challenge of bringing Blanche from the pages of a book to the reality of the stage, and it was magic. I saw myself being successful, and I was successful. I still have a bit of Blanche in me to this day.

What I did for Blanche, you can do for your life. Use constructive daydreaming to define your vision and make that vision real. In that state, you can unlock and unleash the most amazing ideas and creative inspirations,[13] allowing you to evolve to the next levels in your life. This is the way YES! Visions are born!

Now that you know how to daydream using all your senses to help identify your vision take five to ten minutes daily to think about something you would like to occur in the future.

"If you can dream it, you can achieve it." —Zig Ziglar

---

13 Matthijs Baas, Barbara Nevicka, Femke S. Ten Velden, "When Paying Attention Pays off: The Mindfulness Skill Act with Awareness Promotes Creative Idea Generation in Groups." *European Journal of Work and Organizational Psychology*, (2020) 29(4): 619–632.

Step 3: Use Your Inspirations

Do you remember in Chapter 4 when you were tasked with identifying those things that inspire you, those inspirations that motivate you to evolve, change, and grow? It is time to put them to work. It is time to allow your inspirations to propel you forward in the creation of your YES! Vision.

Our inspirations, be they art, music, poetry, or nature, further connect us to our dreams. In elementary school, an opera singer visited my class and sang an operatic aria. At the time, I remember thinking it was absolutely beautiful, and that performance became a constant inspiration throughout my life. Some 30 years later, I sang opera at Carnegie Hall. My inspiration supported my vision of singing, and my vision became my reality.

Step 4: Make Your Goals "Smart"

Every journey begins with that first action step. It is important to move the mental commitment into action. That first action step will be based upon a SMART goal. "SMART" stands for:

1. Specific
2. Measurable
3. Attainable
4. Reasonable
5. Time-sensitive

In other words, each goal must clearly move you toward your desire in a way you can measure, and it must involve reasonable parameters such as timeframes, capabilities, etc.

When working with my clients, I divide SMART goals into SMART Mini and SMART Major goals. Each title denotes the size of the goal you wish to tackle.

SMART Major goals require multiple tasks or actions for their completion. SMART Mini goals are small, specific, and well-defined. SMART Mini goals sometimes comprise parts of SMART Major goals, but they also could be self-standing.

You can use the goals to set milestones along your YES! Journey. As you achieve these goals and evolve as a person, you will gain a richer and deeper understanding of yourself and what moves you, and use that knowledge to set new goals. Your SMART Mini and SMART Major goals can form all of the necessary steps to achieve your YES! Vibrant Vision.

SMART Goals in Action

While I was in the hospital experiencing my transformational moment, I decided that I would diet no more. I had to set attainable goals. After all, I had been living in the extremes: extreme dieting, extreme exercising, in other words, "feast or famine" fitness. When I was in high school, I joined an all-male full-contact karate studio as a way to stay in shape. I had enough bloody noses, split lips, and experiences of having the air knocked out of my lungs to say without hesitation that I was used to the extreme.

When I left the hospital, my first SMART Major goal was to tackle my health challenge. That involved a lot of smaller SMART Mini goals. I pledged to take note of everything I ate and how it made me feel. I was able to design a proper eating plan for myself based upon the effect each food had on my body and on my overall energy level. Likewise, I took a hard look at all my movements and exercises and evaluated how each made me feel. That process gave birth to the YES! System.

Here's another example. Remember my client Monica, the professional nurse/manager with a crazy work schedule? At one point, she set a goal to gain no weight during her family vacation cruise. While it was important that she fully enjoyed all that the cruise offered, Monica's SMART Mini goal was to focus on proper portions. That specific goal helped Monica to lose weight during her trip without even trying. No stress—all fun. By living in a positive mindset, she easily made the proper fitness and nutritional choices while still enjoying the desserts she loved. Imagine losing weight on a cruise!

Monica has maintained her weight loss by continually applying the principles discussed in this book and through her constant commitment to experience greater health.

I gave my recent senior fitness group a SMART Mini goal as part of my YES! Eating program. Their goal/challenge was to reduce their added sugar intake to six teaspoons per day. Achieving that goal enabled many of them to dramatically improve their health to the point where they are no longer being classified as prediabetic. This was a huge achievement, yet, the goal was simple, specific, and attainable.

You can do the same. Keep it small, bite-sized, and doable, and see what is possible.

How to Write a SMART Goal

If you have never written a Smart Major or SMART Mini goal, take a big inhale through your nose and exhale through your mouth, and get ready to get started right now.

Here is an example:

In one year, my daughter and I are planning a hiking trip. Our SMART Major goal is to select the location and the specific date for our hike. We have decided to do a challenging hike with high elevations and multiple hills to traverse. For us, taking this hike is a specific, measurable, attainable, reasonable, and timely goal.

To be able to achieve our SMART Major goal, I need to to set a variety of SMART Mini goals. I will set these SMART Mini goals monthly, weekly, and daily, focusing on continuous improvement of balance, strength, endurance, agility, flexibility, and cardiovascular health to the level necessary to meet the challenge of the hike. For instance:

- **Daily/Weekly** workouts, to include the following per week: Three cardio-based workouts; two strength training workouts; two flexibility-based workouts.
- **Monthly:** Increase the length of each cardio-based workouts; increase the weights and vary the strength-based challenges for each workout; add balance training.

By taking this approach, I will be ready for the chosen hike in one year.

Create Your YES! Vision Statement

Now that you know how to create your goals to advance your dreams, it is time to create your YES! Vision statement.

A vision statement provides a concrete way to reveal your life purpose and see the path toward achieving your long-term desires.

To create your YES! Vision statement, complete the following steps.

1. List the core values you have already reflected on in Chapter 4. (Examples: creativity, family, kindness, respect, innovation, community, etc.)

    _____

    _____

    _____

    _____

    _____

2. Identify what motivates you. Write down the things, thoughts, and/or memories that excite you and give you energy.

    _____

    _____

    _____

    _____

3. Reflect on the people who inspire you. How can you follow in their footsteps, in your own unique way? How would you like to be an inspiration to others? What kinds of actions and qualities would you like to inspire in others?

    _____

    _____

    _____

4. What is your " life"? When you close your eyes and constructively daydream, where do you see yourself and what are you doing? Write it down.

    _____

    _____

    _____

5. Now, let your core values tell you what is most important to you, and let what motivates you illuminate your dreams. Make sure your values are in line with your desires.

    Core Values + Dreams + Inspirations = YES! Vision

    > Core Values
    > + Dreams +
    > Inspirations =
    > YES! Vision

    To create your YES! Vision statement, write down a dream, along with all the senses that you can attach to make it real, while also identifying the inspirations that support it.

    Make sure you know how your dream relates to your Inner Core: your passions, loves, gifts, and talents, as well as your emotional, spiritual, and physical self. Know why achieving this dream is important to you.

For example, the vision for my future has changed over time. When I was in sixth grade, I would watch the legal show, *Perry Mason*, on TV, and I dreamed about becoming a courtroom attorney. I didn't just write down my desire to be a courtroom attorney; I saw myself in the courtroom confronting the witnesses, arguing with defense attorneys, and speaking to the judge.

I heard myself speaking the words and felt my hands slamming the desk for emphasis. In other words, I used my ability to live in the present to fill my daydreams with the specifics that made it feel as if it had already happened. That is the key to creating a vision. That vision propelled me forward to my thirteen-year career as a state and federal prosecutor.

Now, it's your turn.

What is your YES! Vision? Be bold and state it!

_____

_____

_____

_____

_____

_____

6. Now that your YES! Vision is clear, set a SMART goal that moves you toward it. Your goal can be a SMART Major or a SMART Mini goal.

Your YES! Vision SMART goal is:

_____

_____

_____

_____

How will you track your progress on your SMART goal?

_____

_____

_____

_____

Whom can you partner with to hold you accountable for achieving your SMART goal?

_____

_____

_____

Now you are on your way!

Support Your Vision with Affirmations

While on your journey, affirmations will give you the strength to stay the course. An affirmation is a positive statement designed to motivate and encourage yourself to achieve your personal best and reach your personal level of excellence. You have the power to change your emotional state by declaring your positive affirmation with conviction and belief. Create at least one affirmation that supports your desires and repeat it daily.

Examples:

"I love myself and I thank God for my ability to _____ ."

"I am confident and I can _____."

"I will share my gifts with the world by _____."

"I am a Relentless Warrior, ready to do all the work necessary to unleash my full potential."

Now it is your turn.

Write your affirmation and be prepared to state it daily—every morning and every evening. Let your superhero powers shine!

_____

_____

_____

_____

_____

The YES! Take-Away: *Take the necessary steps to live the reality you desire by creating a YES! Vision for the future!*

CHAPTER 7

THE JOY OF AGING— IT IS TRULY JUST A NUMBER

"Aging is not lost youth but a new stage
of opportunity and strength."
—BETTY FRIEDAN

Am I Too Old?

Due in part to the loud voices of many in society, some people think a certain age is "too late to change." I have had clients mistakenly believe that their age dictates the health and condition of their bodies. Have you ever heard someone say, "I'm too old for this," "My body can no longer handle that," "I wish I had done that when I was younger," or, "it's a young man's game"? Society tells us that being older means you are less capable. I really dislike that mindset and those phrases because they are not true. It's time to adopt a framework for thinking about aging that will serve you all the days of your life.

As your coach, I want to bring healing to your brain, your body, and your beliefs and to break the whole negative-habit cycle of words, thoughts, and actions that derail your success.

If you see a handicapped parking space, you think "old." Assisted-living or senior-citizen discounts or privileges may seem like rewards or kindnesses, but they also may operate on the principle that you are incapable. What is most important is that if you begin to take the subtle hint and believe you are incapable, your thoughts become your actions, and your actions reinforce your negative beliefs. As we learned in Chapter 4, negative thoughts can change you and stop you from reaching your goals. It becomes a dangerous mental journey that can alter your perspective on life.

Let's alter that perspective by jumping into aging with a willing brain and body. I call it "Age-Defying Living" (ADL). ADL is the willingness to jump face-forward with momentum into Aging with Grace and Excellence (AGE). When you apply the principles of AGE, possibilities emerge in ways you never imagined.

Living the Age-Defying Life

Honor Your Age

The foundation to living the Age-Defying Life is to honor your TRUE age. I saw a woman being interviewed on TV who, when asked her age, hesitated and then replied, "…Give me a moment; I say so many different ages." Does that sound familiar? The woman was so used to pretending, she had to think about what was actually true. So, I ask you, how old are you? Did you hesitate to answer? Why? Do you see yourself in that woman?

I was forced to confront this issue during the time I was pursuing an acting and singing career. I was up for the title role in the musical *Bessie Smith*. The musical would be performed at a beautiful theatre in New York City, and we had had multiple auditions. We were on the third round of callbacks, and it was now between me and one other singer, who was amazingly talented. Half of the casting team was for me, and half was for the other singer. It was determined that the author of the play would cast the deciding vote.

I will never forget what happened next.

At the time, I was claiming to be seven years younger than I was. I said I was thirty-two, when in fact I was thirty-nine. Casting told me that it had been impossible to pick the better voice, as we were evenly matched. Therefore, they decided to give it to the other singer because (and I quote), "She is closer to the age Bessie Smith was at the time of the musical." They added that I was still "a little young for the part."

Bessie was thirty-nine years old in the musical.

At that moment, I wanted to scream, "I LIED! I AM THIRTY-NINE!" But I didn't. However, that experience reinforced in me the need to be honest about my age and allow myself to Age with Grace and Excellence.

Enjoy the Gifts of Age

Not only should you be "age honest," don't be afraid to state your true age boldly and with excited anticipation. I often refer to it as jumping into aging, which is the opposite of what most people think of doing as they age.

As you shift to the YES! Mindset, never forget all the amazing benefits and gifts that come with aging:

- You are able to think through situations more clearly.
- You no longer worry about peer pressure as a major challenge.
- You have a better understanding of what you like and do not like and are perhaps less fearful of letting others know your needs.
- You have the capacity for deeper, richer understanding and wisdom.
- You have the gift of life experience to uplift yourself and others throughout your life journey.

Aging brings countless jewels to your life. But to fully recognize and add to them, you must be willing to operate within your truth. You will never experience your true desires if you don't allow yourself to embrace and celebrate the true you. I always say that truth elevates all that is positive, while lies reveal the negative within. Live in your truth and elevate your positive nature.

> Truth elevates all that is positive, while lies reveal the negative within.

Age with Grace

Grace has been defined as "elegance or beauty of form, manner, motion, or action; favor or goodwill."[14] Grace is a recognition of

---

14 Dictionary.com, s.v. "Grace," accessed March 20, 2021, https://www.dictionary.com/browse/grace.

the elegance that lies within each of us. It is that elegance that rests within our actions, words, thoughts, and beliefs. When we allow ourselves to hold a state of grace, our inner peace and introspection thrive.

In that state, you will be more capable of tapping into your core self while drowning out those inner and outer negative voices. This state of grace is synonymous with peace, and peace will usher in an internal and external state of wellness that can be life-altering. Are you ready to walk within a peaceful state of wellness? Are you ready to state your truth?

One of my group participants, Jacqueline, recounted living a lifetime of Yo-Yo dieting. She loved sweets and baking and, over the years, allowed her weight to fluctuate by fifty pounds, never returning to her lower weight. Jacqueline referred to her Yo-Yo living as the "Fall back" and was so frustrated that she couldn't gain control over this area of her life. I remember her blaming her age as part of the reason for her extra pounds.

Once Jacqueline learned how to tap into the peaceful mind, age posed no limit and anything was possible. With consistent action, taking "one step at a time," as she put it, Jacqueline found an abundance of power in the YES! Mindset, achieving her goal of losing weight and finding a love of fitness along the way. By incorporating my Yes! Fitness programming requiring daily walks, two to three times per week cardio, and weight-based training, as well as healthy eating habits, Jacqueline's graceful aging continues. She now has "guns" (referring to her arm muscles), and she has found self-motivation and peace of mind.

Age with Excellence

"It's never too late for a new beginning in your life."
—JOYCE MEYER

Aging with Excellence creates an outstanding state of mind. Achieving it requires these four actions:

- Rid yourself of all limiting beliefs and fear of aging.

- Find inspiration in the beauty that surrounds you.

- Constantly challenge the "Three Bs" (Brain, Body, and limiting Beliefs).

- Be inspirational through your daily words and deeds.

No More Limiting Beliefs

In other cultures, seniors are treated as active members of society and family. They do not foster the same self-limiting beliefs. For instance, in Chinatown in New York City, ninety-year-olds are out early in the morning doing Tai-Chi. Why? Because they believe they can still improve their mobility and health with movement. This illustrates that age is not a barrier to participation. The fact is, if you believe that you are too old to improve, you will never improve. You become your beliefs.

Mary, one of my fitness group participants who is also a senior citizen, has this philosophy: "If you stick to it, you can do it."

You are never too old to gain knowledge, to be inspired, to find or have power, or to increase your energy. Make one inspirational step at a time, and see what is possible to you.

Mary had fallen into a temporary funk. Although she had been active earlier in her life, she had drifted into bad eating habits and limited exercise. As a result, her weight increased, and her energy waned. By adopting the principles of ageless living and constant change, Mary dropped seventeen pounds and gained an abundance of energy. Mary's acceptance of the YES! Mindset removed any limits she had previously placed upon herself.

Science Speaks

Regular physical activity and limited sedentary behavior are two of the most important lifestyle strategies to maintain good brain health. Furthermore, physical activity preserves bone and muscle mass and can supply endless sources of energy.[15]

Even though scientific studies support the need for exercise and confirm its positive effects on the body, many of the existing programs geared to the aging population assume they

---

15 Patricia C. Heyn, Mark A. Hirsch, Michele K. York, and Deborah Backus, "Physical Activity Recommendations for the Aging Brain: A Clinician-Patient Guide." *Archives of Physical Medicine and Rehabilitation* June 2016, 97(6): 1045–47. https://doi.org/10.1016/j.apmr.2016.02.003.

lack movement capabilities and are unable to improve. Some programs treat people like they are one step away from the grave—highly condescending! The problem is that there is no "one size fits all approach," and using one will never capture the variation and variety necessary to ignite the participants' commitment and dedication.

To inspire that lifelong commitment, fitness coaches and their participants need a strategy to progress to new achievements, to include variety in executing that strategy, and to understand why and how to move and fuel the body to achieve the main goal of ultimate health. Coaches also need to be skilled in and focused on helping individuals find a love of fitness.

It is my quest to foster a fitness "love story" that differs from one individual to the next. What does yours look like?

Fear No More

"Courage is being afraid but going on anyhow."
—DAN RATHER

Whether to improve your daily living activities, lift things from the floor, go for a walk, go to church, or participate in a marathon, everyone wants to maintain their mobility. No one wants to lose their personal freedoms and become dependent on others. Inactivity has mental and emotional consequences. The loss of your self-confidence and your abilities to do every-day things can lead to depression and anxiety. You will be walking into a mental prison of perpetual fear of inadequacy, and for many, a loss of spontaneity. Your body will begin to work against you.

Physical inactivity will eventually cause you to lose your independence. The less you do, the less you can do. The resulting slow, sluggish, energy-depleted feeling can bring your mind, body, and spirit to the depths of frustration and fear for the future. I have worked with people who have trouble tying their shoes, dressing, walking without pain, or simply getting out of a chair without grunting—but they don't have to be in this situation.

Do you have the energy level you had five years ago? Is your posture as it was at that time?

Right now, even if you don't believe you can improve, that's okay. The YES! System will help you foster your own belief in change— the YES! Mindset. Once I get you to believe in yourself and your abilities, you will start reimagining what aging can be and living your *own* Age-Defying Life!

For me, age has never been a limit in the fitness world. I train with all ages and understand how to push myself to the next level, respecting my brain and my body. I remember once taking fitness training with several military personnel. It was a Tabata Bootcamp certification and it was beyond tough. That day-long training session pushed me further than I thought possible, and I enjoyed every minute. Age did not stand in my way. Don't let it stand in yours.

Constant Challenge for Change

"If you can believe it, the mind can achieve it."
—RONNIE LOTT

To age with excellence, you must constantly challenge the "Three Bs":

- Brain
- Body
- Beliefs

Constantly challenging *all three* continues the forward momentum of your life. As soon as you stop, your momentum stops—your growth, opportunity, development, and possibility stop. Removing your limiting beliefs about age allows you to try new things, reach for new opportunities, and break out of the boxes you have placed yourself within.

We have all heard about the person who retires and then dies soon after. When you retire, your brain, your body, and your belief system can all shut down, and you lose your ability to grow.

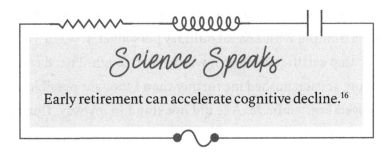

Science Speaks

Early retirement can accelerate cognitive decline.[16]

---

16   Susan Rohwedder and Robert J Willis. "Mental Retirement." *Journal of Economic Perspectives*, February 1, 2010, 24(1): 136. https://doi.org/10.1257/jep.24.1.119.

Challenge Your Brain

To keep the neurons firing and continue to grow the white and grey matter within the brain, you must challenge it on a daily basis. Take a new language class, play a new instrument, learn a new dance, go back to school, or read something challenging and see what is possible.

Science Speaks

The impact of engagement in novel, cognitively challenging activities can improve cognition in older adults. Current results provide some of the first experimental evidence that learning new things and keeping the mind engaged may be important keys to successful cognitive aging.[17]

Challenge Your Body

Your body is your temple, and you are its caretaker. Every day is the day your body can be better, faster, more agile, better balanced, and more energized than the day before.

---

17   D.C. Park, J Lodi-Smith, L. Drew, S. Haber, A. Hebrank, G.N. Bischof, and W. Aamodt, "The Impact of Sustained Engagement on Cognitive Function in Older Adults: The Synapse Project." *Psychological Science*, 2014 25(1): 10.

> Every day is the day your body can be better, faster, more agile, better balanced, and more energized than the day before.

Activate your YES! Mindset and take on a new challenge—use your SMART Mini and Major goals to advance your body's abilities. What additional fitness goal can you add to your day that will give you more capabilities? If you take this challenge, you will be amazed at all you can accomplish. Be an inspiration to yourself and others.

Challenge Your Beliefs

To keep forward momentum, toss your limiting, age-related beliefs into the trash heap with the rest of the negativity from your past. They do not serve you. Then, position the positive beliefs that elevate and illuminate you in a place where they will shine brightly at all times. Those positive beliefs will allow you to become your authentic self. From that center, your God-given talents can flourish and benefit the others around you, as well as yourself.

Marcina was a member of a Mentor/Mentee program I created and implemented through RWJ Beth Israel Medical Center. The purpose of the program was to train individuals from several churches to become certified fitness instructors, helping to infuse a culture of ongoing fitness at the local level. In the beginning, Marcina didn't believe she could pass the exam. Her fear and self-doubt limited her vision. To break through her fear, Marcina focused on her inner strength and Inner Core qualities while remaining dedicated to her studies and willing to take on new challenges as they presented themselves.

Over time, just like Neo in the movie *The Matrix*, she began to believe.

By developing her YES! Mindset, not only did Marcina pass the exam, she also became a certified instructor in multiple fitness modalities. Marcina now teaches classes for RWJ Newark Beth Israel and for a local gym and also runs her own fitness and wellness classes.

She and the other community members who became fitness instructors formed a group called Jointly Fit Together, and they are actively bringing health programming to their churches and to members throughout their communities. Their work is transforming the lives of countless individuals. This group is a force to be reckoned with, and I could not be more proud!

Reflection Exercise

Take a few moments to answer the following questions. Be ready to take action on the answers.

1. What are you willing to do to challenge your brain?

   _____

   _____

2. What are you willing to do to challenge your body?

   _____

   _____

3. What are you willing to do to enhance your YES! Mindset and confront any limiting belief?

_____

_____

Find Inspiration; Become Inspirational

I've mentioned inspiration before when bringing up how to understand your Inner Core and create your YES! Vision. It is the clarity of your vision, along with the inspirations all around , that motivate your actions and provide you with unlimited strength. Inspiration strengthens your resolve to break down the barriers that separate you from your dreams. Inspiration shows you what is possible and makes you want to accomplish new things. It challenges you as well as strengthens you.

Seek inspiration everywhere—in music, dance, art, literature, sports, individual accomplishments, and nature, to name a few sources. Be aware, be intentional, and let that which inspires you guide you toward inspiring others.

Individuals all over the world are breaking down barriers and opening pathways every day, inspiring us to do more than we ever thought possible. These people have lived by the phrase, "Nothing is impossible," and we can learn from them.

Charles Eugster

At the age of sixty-three, retired dental surgeon Charles Eugster rekindled a love of competitive rowing he'd neglected for most of his adult life. He took up bodybuilding at eighty-seven. And when he was ninety-five, he started sprinting for the first time in his life, becoming World Champion at the 200m indoor and the 400m outdoor. He was a world record-holder for his age group in a number of sports with forty gold medals for World Masters Rowing.[18]

Betty Reid Soskin

Ninety-nine-year-old Betty Reid Soskin is the oldest serving ranger for the United States National Park Service. Betty conducts park tours and serves as an interpreter, explaining the park's purpose, history, various sites, and museum collections to park visitors.

When commenting on her life in 2015 at the age of 93, she wrote, "Wish I'd had confidence when the 'young Betty' needed it to navigate through the hazards of everyday life on the planet. But maybe I'm better able to benefit from having it now—when I have the maturity to value it and the audacity to wield it for those things held dear."[19]

Frances Woofenden

Frances Woofenden has collected a small mountain of awards and medals after getting started in waterskiing at the age of fifty. At eighty-one, Frances still goes waterskiing five days a week on the lakes near her home.[20]

---

18   "Record-breaking veteran spints sensation Charles Eugster dies aged 97." Athleticsweekly.com, accessed March 29th, 2021. https://athleticsweekly.com/ athletics-news/record-breaking-veteran-sprints-sensation-charles-eugster-dies-97-60363/

19   https://en.wikipedia.org/wiki/Betty_Reid_Soskin; Betty Reid Soskin, "I'm 99, And the Oldest Park Ranger in America." Newsweek, October 11, 2020, page 1.

20   "Frances Woofenden," pinterest.com, accessed March 29, 2021, https://www.pinterest. com.au/pin/386957792988558148/, https://www.flickr.com/photos/35328881@ N06/3272799743/

Johanna Quaas

At eighty-eight years old, German native Johanna Quaas is the oldest active gymnast in the world. Quaas, born in 1925, started doing gymnastics at an early age and participated in her first competition in 1934. Eighty years later, she's still competing, and her participation in the Turnier der Meister in Cottbus, Germany, in 2012 earned her an entry in *The Guinness Book of World Records* as the oldest gymnast in the world. The grandmother and mother of three has been married to Gerhard Quaas, a gymnastics coach, for more than fifty years.[21]

Sister Madonna Bruder

An Ironman competition involves completing—in one day—a 2.4-mile swim, a 112-mile bike, and a 26.2-mile run (a marathon). This is difficult enough in your prime, but Sister Madonna Bruder, a Catholic nun, has done over forty-five of these races and continues to compete at age eighty-six.[22]

Yuichiro Miura

Mount Everest is the tallest mountain in the world, and climbing it is a dangerous, grueling undertaking. However, in 2014,

21   Nicol Natale, "Watch the World's Oldest Gymnast Crush a Seriously Impressive Routine in Viral Video." December 23, 2020, page 1. https://www.prevention.com/fitness/a35056966/johanna-quaas-gymnastics-video-twitter/

22   Kevin Mackinnon, "Sister Madonna Buder turns 90 today." Triathlon Magazine Canada, July 24, 2020, page 1. https://triathlonmagazine.ca/personalities/sister-madonna-buder-turns-90-today/

Japanese climber Yuichiro Miura, born in 1932, became the oldest person to reach the summit—and it was his third time.[23]

Lisa Charles

At twenty-four years of age, I entered the practice of law as a state prosecutor, later becoming a federal prosecutor. I had the chance to prosecute every type of crime, and I enjoyed the courtroom for many years. I won every federal case. I left law to pursue a singing and acting career. I sang jazz, Broadway, and opera and had the chance to do a one-woman show, sing in concerts, and perform in many Off-Broadway productions. I played Blanche in *A Streetcar Named Desire* for the African Globe Theater and sang at Carnegie Hall. After experiencing a vocal injury, I entered the fitness/wellness field as an instructor, trainer, health coach, and later as a health and wellness consultant and a wellness presenter.

Now, at fifty-eight, I am the CEO of Embrace Your Fitness, LLC and am the fitness/wellness research coordinator for the Rutgers University Aging & Brain Health Alliance.

And I am now an author![24]

Envision Your Own Story

All right; now, it's your turn! You get to write your own future story about how you lived an Age-Defying Life. What do you

---

23 "Japanese climber Yuichiro Miura, 86, to 'hang on to the last' in summit attempt of Argentina's Mount Aconcagua." japantimes.co.jp, accessed March 29, 2021, page 1. https://www.japantimes.co.jp/news/2018/12/04/national/japanese-climber-yuichiro-miura-86-hang-last-bid-scale-argentinas-mount-aconcagua/

24 https://vimeo.com/530962967

want that story to be? Your story will continue to evolve over the years, so let's look at the short-term story and the long-term story.

1. What will your story be six months from now? Write it in the past tense as if it's already happened.

    _____

    _____

    _____

    _____

2. What will your story be in ten years? Again, write it in the past tense. Really envision your future accomplishments as if you have already achieved them.

    _____

    _____

    _____

    _____

I am excited—how about you?

The YES! Take-Away: *Jump into your age and enjoy an Age-Defying Life!*

CHAPTER 8

JUST BREATHE—THE H2H OF BREATH

Finding Your Breath

When I was young, I used to have this nightmare of being trapped underground with a limited supply of oxygen. I would wake up gasping for air, full of fear, with one thought and one thought only: Just breathe!

One cannot overestimate the power of breath. It is said that there exists a "rule of threes" relating to the nature of what our bodies need: we can only go three weeks without food, three days without water, and three minutes without oxygen. Our reliance on oxygen, defined in terms of only minutes, shows that our need for it is most dire.

I liken breath to an internal mega-power source that can unleash unlimited possibilities in the brain's capacity to process information and the body's ability to react. You can use your breath as a tool to help move your brain into a state of complete focus, where creativity and imagination can thrive, or into a state of absolute relaxation, reducing stress and anxiety to enable peace and calm.

> *"Breathe. Let go. And remind yourself that this very moment is the only one you know you have for sure."*
> —OPRAH WINFREY

Think of each breath as a vehicle to improve concentration and productivity, to enhance sleep and emotional stability, and to release harmful byproducts and toxins from your system. In fact, your breath can improve respiration and cardiovascular function, decrease stress, and improve your mental and physical health.[25] *It is your Life Force.*

Your every breath is also a gateway to identifying your true desire and illuminating the pathway to its realization. You have immense power, yet it lies dormant inside you, as it does within many, until you activate it.

Despite this incredible power that rests inside each of us, poor breathing habits plague many, affecting their health and exposing them to a variety of maladies. Breath is life, and it is needed to advance every function within the body.

Shallow, chest breathing inhibits the advancement of the brain-body connection as it prevents the ability of oxygen to reach and nourish all the body's cells. Without tapping that

---

25 A.V. Turankar, S Jain, S. B. Patel, S. R. Sinha, A. D. Joshi, B. N. Vallish, P. R. Mane, and S.A. Turankar. "Effects of Slow Breathing Exercise on Cardiovascular Functions, Pulmonary Functions & Galvanic Skin Resistance in Healthy Human Volunteers—a Pilot Study." n.d., 1. https://pubmed.ncbi.nlm.nih.gov/23760377/.

internal power source through focused breathwork, the ability to truly thrive within the brain-body connection will elude you.

Science Speaks

Long-term shallow breathing can lead to stress, which is a common risk factor in 75 to 90 percent of all human diseases.[26] "Breathing becomes dysfunctional when the person is unable to breathe efficiently or when breathing is inappropriate, unhelpful, or inefficient in responding to environmental conditions and the changing needs of the individual. Impairment of the functions of breathing affects people's lives, creating symptoms and compromising health."[27]

The Power of Focused Breath
Focused breath, which allows you to tap into that internal power source, brings you into the present, and basking in the present

26 Yun-Zi Liu, Yun-Xia Wang, and Chun-Lei Jiang. "Inflammation: the common pathway of stress-related diseases." *Frontiers in Human Neuroscience* (2017) 11: 316.

27 Courtney Rosalba. "The Functions of Breathing and Its Dysfunctions and Their Relationship to Breathing Therapy." *International Journal of Osteopathic Medicine*, September 2009, 12(3): 78–85. https://doi.org/10.1016/j.ijosm.2009.04.002.

allows true creativity to flow. With focus, you can regain and reclaim the breathing process that you were born with.

Proper breathing supplies your body with the right amount of oxygen to replenish your brain and other vital organs with essential nutrients. Breathing helps improve your digestion, increase your metabolism, and improve your overall blood flow.

Your cardiopulmonary system helps transport those nutrients through your circulatory system to each and every cell of your body while helping to remove toxins from your system. Researchers also hypothesize that exhaling helps eliminate fat molecules from our bodies. That's right—fat molecules! In other words, your breath helps to keep what is good for you, while clearing out what is bad.

As babies, we all took deep, relaxing breaths from our abdomens. If you watch a baby sleep, you will see the gentle rise and fall of its belly. It is so beautiful and peaceful to witness. But as we get older, we change our breathing patterns. Partly due to ongoing stress and poor habits, our formerly deep, belly-level inhalations and exhalations shrink into shallow, short, chest / thoracic breaths.

It is estimated that on average, we take twelve to eighteen breaths per minute, which is 18,000–26,000 per day when we only need six breaths per minute to meet our bodies' needs.[28] Stress can lead to shallow breathing, and this breathing pattern

---

28 Marc A. Russo, Danielle M. Santarelli, and Dean O'Rourke. "The Physiological Effects of Slow Breathing in the Healthy Human." *Breathe*, December 2017, 13(4): 306. https://doi.org/10.1183/20734735.009817.

can increase stress within the body. This stress robs you of your ability to operate at an optimum level—and cheats you of your ability to tune into and achieve your goals. You become a breathing "survivor" as opposed to a breathing "thriver," and if you are not careful, you may fall back into that "mindless-zombie" existence.

By being mindful of your breathing and consciously using it to thwart stress—using the YES! Breathing approach—you can help assure the advancement of your health and your brain-body wellness.

The Power of YES! Breathwork

You can pair your YES! Breathwork with other types of skills you've already learned so as to achieve even greater results. Let's start by doing the breath exercise shown in the "Five Breaths to Better Focus". When your breath is slow, deep, and focused, you can begin to use each breath to transition and transform.

For instance, you can engage in focused, constructive

Five Breaths to Better Focus

To experience focused breath:

1. Sit at the edge of a chair, resting your forearms gently on your thighs.

2. Roll your shoulders back and down so that your chest will lift.

3. In that position, take a long, cleansing breath in through your nose, and exhale through your mouth.

4. Repeat 5 times. You should begin to experience the sense of calm that focused breathing can bring.

To get the most out of this exercise, try making it a SMART Mini goal and use it to replace one of your undesired mental, physical, or emotional habits.

daydreaming, as discussed in Chapter 4, using each cleansing breath to bring life, details, colors, texture, and new ideas to your vision. Allow those breaths to shape your vision more clearly and fuel it with greater power.

During my singing career, I often used the power of YES! Breathwork to fully envision myself performing at shows before they took place. During those breath-enriched daydreams, I would see musical changes or unique phraseology that I would then bring to life during performances. I remember a show I created called *The Poetry of Music*. It combined the spoken word with a variety of Negro spirituals. I spent time allowing my breath and its connection with my creative internal force to help guide me emotionally and visually to see and feel the connection between each poem and each musical piece selected. I allowed that process to help me envision how to tell the story in a truthful, impactful, and memorable manner.

Let your breath help you make new discoveries that you never thought possible. You may be one breath away from making a revelation that can change the direction of your life—or someone else's, through your inspiration.

Breathe Through the Tough Times

In your darkest moments, when all around is negative, you can use your breath as a vehicle to take you back into the light. With each deep, rich, diaphragmatic breath, you can bring forth positive thoughts and a renewed state of calm. With your enhanced brain-body connection through the YES! System, each calming breath will help the brain release neurochemicals to dissolve stress, reduce pain, boost cognition, and increase your feeling of trust and inner peace.

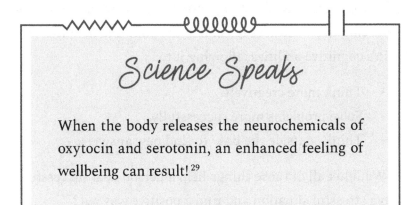

Science Speaks

When the body releases the neurochemicals of oxytocin and serotonin, an enhanced feeling of wellbeing can result! [29]

You can also use focused breath to power through emotional challenges when dealing with difficult issues by pairing it with other exercises in this book. Think about those moments, as addressed in Chapter 3, when you took on your internal defeaters—those negative, recurring, destructive thoughts that held sway over your mind. When you are purposely allowing your negative thoughts to play out so you can identify their lies, untruths, and misrepresentations, you can use deep diaphragmatic breaths to remain grounded and focused.

Imagine someone who has lost their job, with a family who depends on them and limited money in the bank. The reality of such a loss has the potential to engulf that person's every thought

29   Grace Alessi, MD, "The Four Body-Manufactured Chemicals That Affect Happiness, Balanced Well-Being." *Healthcare*, December 21, 2018, 1.

and sink them into the depths of sadness, disappointment, and fear. Whereas the power of breath will not solve the underlining challenge, using deep, diaphragmatic breathing in such moments of extreme stress releases tension in the body and heightens the brain's cognitive abilities, allowing it to:

- Think more creatively.
- Solve problems more successfully.
- Think "outside the box" to find new answers.

Wouldn't all of those things help a person deal successfully with a stressful situation and find a positive way out?

Even in those times when Yo-Yo habits threaten to return, focused breath can bring you back to your authentic self, reinstating your true desires so the negative thought spiral cannot lead you back into destructive actions.

During my current health groups, I lead participants through slow/focused breathing sessions to calm the mind, lift up the spirit, and achieve peace.

Breathe for Better Health

The beauty of focused breathing lies in the multiple ways it can transform your health. Believe it or not, in addition to helping you de-stress and induce a state of calm, something so simple as deep breathing can help you to sleep, to make better food choices, to lose weight, and to exercise with improved muscle and overall body efficiency.

One of the key components of the YES! System is to mindfully *experience* the wonders of deep, slow, rich diaphragmatic breaths. With each focused breath, you have the power of healing and self-discovery. Breathe and elevate your passions; breathe and elevate your dreams; breathe and elevate your goals.

Are you ready to experience what focused breath can do for you?

Exercise: Three-Minute Wake-Up Breath

In three minutes, you can clear your mental fog and give your body a wake-up call. Try it now, and record your experience in the lines below:

- Breathe in through your nose and feel your belly expanding.

- Hold that breath for three seconds.

- Blow the air out through your mouth until all air is out of your belly.

- Repeat five times, slowing down the exhalation each time.

- On the sixth exhalation, at the end, gently close your lips and hold your breath for the count of ten to twenty. Take in a deep breath, and exhale.

- Resume normal breathing.

Record your experience. Was it difficult? Easy? How did you feel before and after?

_____

_____

_____

_____

_____

The YES! Take-Away: *Commit to daily breathing exercises and let the power of your breath empower you—Brain, Body, and Spirit.*

CHAPTER 9

THE H2H: HEALTHY HEALING FUEL HABITS

With your commitment to the YES! Mindset, you have begun to advance your brain-body connection and are now positioned to experience the full benefits that healthy healing fueling/ eating habits can bring. You have Committed—now is the time to Do!

> You are a reflection of not only what you choose to eat, but also how you choose to move.

When you fuel your body, you fuel your brain, and when you move your body to enhance your muscles, that movement enhances your brain. My mom used to say, "You are what you eat," and she was partially correct. You are a reflection of not only what you choose to eat, but also how you choose to move. The choices you make either help create an environment bringing internal peace, health, and wellness, or one of stress, sickness, and disease.

You cannot control all aspects of your health, but the YES! System is designed to help you choose wisely regarding those factors that you do control.

The fueling process affects every cell of your body. Each cell needs proper nutrients to function, and you rely upon healthy digestive and cardiovascular systems to accommodate your body's needs.

Fueling habits that bring about health and healing rely on a healthy gut. Your gut and your brain are closely linked. When the microbiome, or the bacteria that is a part of your gut, is unhealthy, your brain will likely be unhealthy. This unhealthy state could lead to emotional instability, depression, mental confusion, and a breakdown of physical abilities.[30]

Additionally, the way in which you eat and the state of your body when you eat can both directly impact the health of your brain and body. Stress, poor food choices, and poor eating habits can limit your ability to experience full wellness. The YES! System is meant to help you align your habits with your goals to reduce your stress and achieve better balance throughout your life, including your general health and wellness.

By taking ownership of all aspects of fueling your body, you take a crucial step forward toward furthering your YES! Journey, enhancing the state of your brain-body connectivity.

Are you ready to take a big step forward and do it now?

---

30 M. Carabotti, A. Scirocco, M. Maselli, and C. Severi, "The Gut-Brain Axis: Interactions Between Enteric Microbiota, Central and Enteric Nervous Systems." *Annal of Gastroenterology*, 2015, 28(2): 203–209. https://www.ncbi.nlm.nih.gov/pmc/articles/PMC4367209/

Four Fueling Habits Designed to Transform Your Health

1. The Kitchen Is Closed

I distinctly remember a time when, as a child, I snuck downstairs into the kitchen late at night to grab a snack. From a distance, my mom yelled, "The kitchen is closed!" My mom wanted us to give our bodies a chance to digest our food between dinner and breakfast, when we would resume our eating routine. It was her attempt to give us children a healthy habit, but at the time, I was just greatly disappointed. To this day, those words ring in my mind. And as a health coach, though I'm not standing in their kitchens, I make those words ring in the ears of all my clients!

What is It?

"The Kitchen Is Closed" is my term for a form of intermittent fasting. With intermittent fasting, you time meals on a schedule that allows for periods of fasting and periods of fueling. This process elicits an evolutionary cellular response that can improve glucose regulation, increase stress resistance, and suppress inflammation. In other words, intermittent fasting helps the body function more efficiently and protect its cells.

During fasting periods, cells are protected against oxidative and metabolic stress, and during feeding periods, cells engage in tissue growth and plasticity. Intermittent fasting can also reverse aging and disease processes while bolstering mental and physical performance.[31]

---

31   Andreas von Bubnoff, "The When of Eating: The Science Behind Intermittent Fasting." *Knowable Magazine*, January 29, 2021, 17.

How to Do It

The "Kitchen Is Closed" method requires you to set a time to stop eating for the evening. Your dinnertime is your final fueling period for the evening. Once finished, you will not resume eating until a minimum of twelve hours later. That will be your breakfast when you literally "break the fast."

The amount of fasting time can be twelve, sixteen, twenty, or even twenty-four hours. You can vary the times and thus ultimately the response your body will experience.

Making it Work

The "Kitchen Is Closed" is a key component of the wellness programming I design and coordinate. I challenged my senior group to observe this rule for one week, and the results were tremendous. Of the twenty-five individuals who took part in the challenge, all reported increased energy, fifteen experienced weight loss, and all reported being able to sleep more soundly. It works for me, it worked for my groups, and now it can work for you.

2. Feel the Fuel

At my "Ah-ha" moment in the hospital, when I decided I was ready to experience lasting change and was committed to never dieting again, I decided to use my brain and my body to figure it out. I did not have a roadmap, nor did I know the exact steps that I would take. I was, however, committed to a discovery process, and I created the "Feel the Fuel" process to begin that journey.

What is It?

"Feel the Fuel" is the process of evaluating the impact each food you consume has on your body. Each food group, each spice and herb, has a unique texture and flavor and will affect each individual's body differently. This step-by-step process will provide invaluable information as you determine the best ways to fuel your body.

How to Do It

As I mentioned, I began this process shortly after leaving the hospital, after dealing with an intestinal infection. While in the hospital, I learned that I weighed north of two hundred pounds. I left the hospital determined to make a difference in my health.

First, I kept a journal of both the food and beverages that I consumed. I used the "Kitchen Is Closed" practice to reset my body and prepare myself for this new health journey.

Then, **before every meal**, I asked:

- Is this what I want?
- Will this advance my health?
- Is there a better choice?

And after each meal, I asked:

- How did the food make me feel?
- Am I satisfied—**not full?**

Making it Work

By being mindfully engaged in the fueling process, I created a strong relationship between my brain and my body. The communication between my gut and my brain enabled me to gain a deep understanding of that internal relationship, which then helped me to make better food choices. Not only did I feel better and have more energy, but my digestion and elimination improved as well.

As a result, meal by meal, day by day, and month by month, the healthy choices I made led to a seventy-seven-pound weight loss and the strength of knowing nothing was impossible for me. I know that I can do anything I set my mind and heart to. That empowering knowledge formed the core essence of the YES! System.

3. Slow it Down

What is It?

This Healthy Healing Habit is exactly what it says. Slow down the timing of your food intake. This habit will strongly enhance your brain-body connection by allowing the Vagus nerve, the connective nerve between your gut and your brain, to communicate true sensations of hunger and satisfaction. This communication will lead to natural, non-stressful portion control. You will just automatically know when to eat and when to stop eating if you allow your gut to let you know when you are truly hungry and when you are satisfied.

How to Do It

The best way to apply this habit is to do the following three things:

- Chew each bite of food until it is almost dissolved.

- Focus on tasting, savoring the flavor of, and thoroughly enjoying each morsel you consume.

- Apply the 20/10 Rule: Take twenty minutes to eat each meal, and eat with no distractions. Then take a ten-minute walk after your last meal of the day. That ten-minute walk will not only help improve your fitness but will also be a digestion booster!

Making it Work

Today, I want you to apply this habit to your fueling process. Treat yourself as a King or Queen and take the time to cherish each bite of food. Try to taste each spice and flavor that enters your mouth and engage in savoring the experience. Do this for a minimum of five chews.

To really make the point of this experience, I had the participants in one of my groups take out their best china and silverware and have an elegant virtual lunch. Maybe that will not work every day, but it certainly helps change the mindset about how we fuel our bodies.

4. Drink the Air and the Water

What is It?

The brain and the body need oxygen and water to survive. There are no words that can adequately express the importance of the effects hydration and breathing have on every cell of the body.

This habit uses breath to improve your food-fueling and digestive processes by enhancing the communication between your gut and your brain.

- Breath—fat loss happens through exhalation

- Water—water's effect on digestion and body temperature regulation is crucial as we are made mostly of water.

How to Do It
This simple tip pays big dividends.

- Take five diaphragmatic breaths before each meal to ensure that you are hungry and not simply lacking sufficient oxygen.

- Drink eight to ten ounces of water before each meal to make sure you are not confusing thirst with hunger.

Sometimes the small changes make a large difference in our ability to transform.

Making it Work
Daily commitment is essential to experiencing lasting success. Take time to practice your breathing techniques as set forth in earlier chapters, and make sure you take your five cleansing breaths and drink your water before every meal and every snack.

Science Speaks

You can significantly reduce cognitive decline by consuming two or more daily servings of vegetables, with the strongest association observed with six or more servings weekly of green leafy and other vegetables.[32]

The Yes! Take-Away: *Small habits can bring about big changes!*

32   MC Morris, DA Evans, CC Tangney, JL Bienias, and RS Wilson, "Associations of Vegetable and Fruit Consumption with Age-Related Cognitive Change." *Neurology*, 2006, 67 (8):1011. https://n.neurology.org/content/67/8/1370.full

CHAPTER 10

THE H2H: HEALTHY HEALING FIT HABITS

"Excellence is an art won by training and habituation...
Excellence, then, is not an act but a habit."
—WILL DURANT

The Key: Brain-Body Connectivity

Fitness of the brain and the body require consistent actions that promote internal and external connectivity. That connectivity advances overall body awareness and internal strength while promoting the positive outlook that exemplifies the YES! Mindset. Whether it is the brain's signal to each muscle as you perform activities of daily living, such as walking, climbing, lifting, pushing, or pulling, or the release of hormones and chemicals to support sleeping, eating, thinking, the brain-body connection is essential to healthy living.

The following Healthy Healing Fit Habits advance that connectivity by improving posture and sleep quality, while increasing the ability to feel and fire up physical movements to advance your YES! Body.

1. Posture is King and Queen

> *"Posture is the most overlooked key to better health."*
> —ROBERT COOPER

How would you like to grow an instant inch? How would you like to shrink your abdomen a half-inch in a matter of moments? Does that even sound possible? The truth is, when you exercise proper posture, you can change your appearance instantly and help optimize your breathing and your body's circulatory system.

What is It?

Posture is the body's ability to maintain balance, alignment, and proper motion. Specifically, balance refers to the body's ability to maintain the line of gravity within the base of support so it can remain upright. Alignment is how the head, shoulders, spine, hips, knees, and ankles relate to and line up with each other.

Several researchers have suggested that maintaining correct posture and breathing habits could be the most important factor in promoting health and energy.[33]

---

33 Cari Nierenberg,"Sit Up Straight! How Good Posture Benefits Your Health." *Live Science,* April 04, 2016.

In addition to balance and alignment, proper posture has the ability to increase lung capacity, overall energy, and self-confidence while decreasing stress on the back and joints and removing tension in the neck and shoulders. Its importance cannot be overestimated.

Good posture is essential in everything from walking across the room to going up and down the stairs, rising out of a chair, or carrying heavy packages. It can enhance your quality of life and improve your ability to perform everyday activities. Given its importance to the health of multiple areas within the body, focus on proper posture is essential.[34]

How to Do It

The YES! System has you practice proper posture (the "Double P") daily. Posture is a frame from which your muscles, lungs, organs, etc., live and function. If you have a weak frame, it can collapse. Gravity never quits, so it is important to strengthen your frame.

Follow the listed steps and begin to experience the many benefits the Double P can provide. Don't worry about being perfect—just be consistent.

---

34 The Ohio State University. "Body Posture Affects Confidence In Your Own Thoughts, Study Finds." ScienceDaily, October 5, 2009.

WHILE SITTING AT A DESK:

- Keep your feet on the floor.

- Don't cross your legs. Your ankles should be directly in front of your knees, keeping a small gap between them.

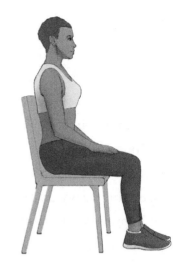

- Your knees should be at or below the level of your hips.

- Relax your shoulders and keep your forearms parallel to the ground.

- Remove any tension from the neck and create a distance from your ears to your shoulders.

WHEN STANDING:

- Stand straight, keeping your knees slightly bent and your gaze straight ahead.

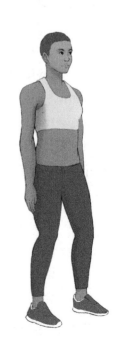

- Keep a neutral spine.

- Center your body's weight over your feet and ground your stance into the floor.

- Keep your feet about shoulder/hip width apart.

- Roll your shoulders to the back and down engaging the muscles of your shoulder blades.

- Let your arms hang down the sides of the body.

- Remove any tension from the neck and create a distance from your ears to your shoulders.[35]

It is essential that you claim your Royalty status as the King or Queen of your stature. I have never seen Queen Elizabeth slumped over or looking down at the ground as she walks, sits, or stands.

Making it Work

As a health coach and trainer, I instruct every client and every fitness group as to how they can improve posture by focusing on specific balancing exercises. These exercises are designed to increase muscle strength while improving muscle coordination and flexibility. Achieving this is key to the YES! System. One of these, the plank, is described in #3, Be "Breathe Fit," below. You can also find more movement-oriented exercises at www.YesCoachLisa.com/Inspirations.

However, in addition to recommending specific exercises, I always stress the importance of continually focusing on posture during all daily activities of living. You can actually practice and

---

35   American Chiropractic Association, "Maintaining Good Posture." accessed March 20, 2021, https://www.acatoday.org/Patients/Health-Wellness-Information/Posture.

improve your posture every minute of your day if you make it a priority. With all of its benefits, you have a lot to gain—so why not give it a try?

My client Rosie came to me from the hospital system. She was an employee with a heavy client caseload and a crazy work schedule. As part of her work, she was often in a forward-leaning position. At the beginning of our work together, Rosie had the habit of walking slightly bent over, with her gaze downward.

We focused our initial training on improving her posture and increasing her core strength, both of which are fundamental to the YES! System. By working on her balance, back and chest muscles, and core strength, we were able to enhance Rosie's brain-body connection. Rosie began to *feel* when her posture was out of alignment—she didn't need someone to tell her or to see it in a mirror. Self-awareness is a key step toward igniting change.

She achieved her improved brain-body connection through a series of single-leg exercises and plank holds. While performing each exercise, Rosie would focus on the feeling of each engaged muscle. This laser focus led Rosie to internally understand more deeply which muscles actually held her posture during each exercise. Through our work, Rosie was able to experience a taller, more upright posture and a forward-lifted gaze. She now carries herself like Royalty.

As I tell all my trainees, you are truly the King or Queen of your personal YES! Journey. Be aware of and demonstrate your Royalty status at all times—you never know when I may spot you on the street.

2. Get "Sleep-Fit"

To be YES! Body-fit, you must be "sleep fit." An adult body needs seven to nine hours of sleep to function at its true capacity. If you are meeting that requirement, you are sleep-fit. If you are not getting the required sleep, your body is suffering, even though you may not feel it. Therefore, it's vital to honor sleep's importance and commit to making the changes necessary to do so.

What Is It?

We all know what sleep is, but do you know its myriad benefits? Sleep restores the entire body and aids in cellular recuperation. Namely, it aids in muscle growth and tissue repair while boosting the body's overall immune system.[36] Poor sleep can affect your gut microbiome, which can cause inflammation, insulin sensitivity, and obesity.

A cleansing process occurs in the brain during deep sleep.[37] The brain cells can shrink in size by about 30 percent. With all that space around your neurons, various metabolic byproducts and toxins get cleared and washed out through the cerebral spinal fluid. This can only occur when you experience restorative sleep. If you do not, you may experience higher instances of stress, poor

---

36   https://www.ninds.nih.gov/Disorders/Patient-Caregiver-Education/Understanding-Sleep D. Foley, S. Ancoli-Israel, P. Britz, and J. Walsh, "Sleep Disturbances and Chronic Disease in Older Adults: Results of the 2003 National Sleep Foundation Sleep in America Survey." *J Psychosom Res* 2004 56: 497–502.

37   Victoria Frankel, "The Gut Microbiome and Sleep: 3 Ways Your Gut Can Impact Your Sleeping Patterns." Viome, December 15, 2019, p.1-2. https://www.viome.com/blog/3-ways-your-gut-microbiome-can-impact-sleep

concentration, an increased risk of dementia, and an overall lack of energy. Lack of sleep can make even the *simplest* physical fitness routine an insurmountable challenge.

How to Do It

The key to experiencing the benefits of restorative sleep lies in two main factors: Your sleep rituals and your sleep environment.

Sleep rituals are the routines you do before going to bed. When done with regularity, sleep rituals can train the brain to ready the body for sleep. Essentially, each step in your ritual will progressively lead to a deeper state of relaxation.

Examples of sleep rituals:

- **Impose a daily bedtime** at the same time each day.

- **Before bedtime, drink a cup of hot green tea.** Green tea contains amino acids that can help de-stress.

- **Take an evening hot bath** or shower.

- **Do a five-to-ten-minute evening stretch** with deep breathing.

- **Turn off all electronics** at least thirty minutes before your bedtime.

These rituals signal your body to relax and prepare for sleep. Your rituals can also include meditation, listening to calming music, or taking a short, relaxing walk. Be creative. Just be dedicated to establishing routines that set you up for sleep success.

Sleep environment refers to the place where you sleep. This area should support deep, restorative sleep.

Some tips for creating a positive sleep environment include:

- **Keep it dark.** A dark room fosters deep sleep.

- **Keep it quiet.** No television, no computers, tablets, or cell-phones — no noise. Sleep in a silent environment allows for the four sleep cycles to take place. Each step is critical to assuring the relaxation and the elimination of toxins from the body.

- **Keep it cool.** Science shows that a cool environment fosters non-disruptive sleep.

- **Keep it comfortable.** Invest in a mattress, sheets, comforter, and pillow that will invite deep sleep.

- **Keep it tidy.** A cluttered room may lead to a cluttered mind.

- **Lose the blue.** In addition to eliminating anything that can create a noisy environment, it is essential that you eliminate all devices that emanate a blue light. These include the TV, cellphones, laptops, and tablets. Science has shown that this light disrupts sleep, preventing the brain and body from experiencing the sleep cycles that foster deep relaxation and the elimination of toxins. [38]

---

38 "Beware of Blue Light Before Sleep." Brighamhealthhub.org, accessed March 29, 2021, https://brighamhealthhub.org/beware-of-blue-light-before-sleep/.

I want my body to rid itself of all toxins—how about you? Take the steps and approach sleep as you do any other exercise you wish to perfect.

Making it Work

Sleep fitness is a key component of the YES! System because of the energy, clarity, agility, and coordination it brings to daily movement. Since insufficient sleep affects the body's ability to convert calories into the energy needed to exercise efficiently, as a coach and trainer, I want my clients to enhance their sleep.

You, too, can experience the multiple benefits that a good night's sleep can provide. Just take this Sleep Fit Challenge that I give to all my participants: Today, challenge yourself to create sleep rituals and a sleep environment that will help advance your brain health. Doing so will give you a boost of physical energy and mental clarity that will support your YES! Journey. The challenge is yours!!

Sleep is not only essential in maintaining a healthy immune system, body temperature, and blood pressure; sleeplessness can increase instances of heart attacks and can lead to obesity, diabetes and dementia.[39]

---

39 D. Foley D, Ancoli-Israel S, Britz P, Walsh J. "Sleep disturbances and chronic disease in older adults: results of the 2003 National Sleep Foundation Sleep in America Survey." J Psychosom Res 2004; 56: 497–502.

3. Be "Breath Fit"

What is It?

As you learned earlier, breath is the gateway to unlocking your internal power source. When you harness that power, it can transform every muscle in your body. The key is to use your oxygen inhalation and CO_2 exhalation as a mechanism for igniting more of your muscle fibers while reinforcing the connection between those fibers and your brain.

This is top-down, inside-out fitness.

How to Do It

Breath fitness is based upon mastering the two components that make up the internal mechanisms that allow you to breathe. The first component is the diaphragm, which draws air in and expands and fills the pump. The second component consists of the deep core muscles (called the Transversus Abdominis) that push the air out, emptying the lungs as the diaphragm relaxes and recoils. I call this mechanism the Vitality Pump, and it is your power source.

To engage or power up your Vitality Pump, take the following steps:

- Inhale through your nose, filtering the air, and allow your belly to expand as if you are smelling a flower.

- Exhale through your mouth with pursed lips and closed teeth. Make a 'Ph' or 'S' sound as you exhale, which will engage your core muscles. Feel the sound as you exhale.
- With each breath, add length to your exhalation.

While activating your Vitality Pump, you should feel the rise and fall of your abdomen, whether you are upright or lying down. This is breathing the way you did when you were born. Watch a baby breathe. As they inhale, their entire belly expands, and as they exhale, everything contracts. To optimize your Vitality Pump, commit to five minutes of this type of focused breathing daily.

There is a direct connection between core stabilization and the pursed-lip breathing (PLB) technique with prolonged exhalation used in the exercise above. PLB is a technique that allows people to control their oxygenation and ventilation.

Feel the tightening of your abdominal muscles as they fall inward during your pursed-lip exhalation. Science has proven that you can achieve more intensive activation of the core muscles with PLB prolonged exhalation.[40] *That's your untapped internal power source!!*

Making it Work

This is your pathway to truly feeling your muscles. To practice this power-enhancing method, apply it to the plank exercise, which happens to be one of my favorites!

---

40 Merrithew, "The Basic Principles: Breathing." accessed March 29, 2021, https://www.merrithew.com/stott-pilates/warmup/en/principles/breathing.

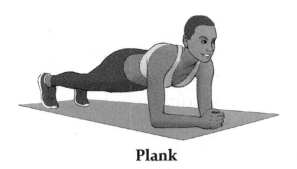

Plank

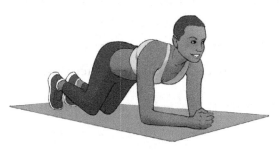

Plank with Knee

The Plank

Begin on your stomach, placing your hands and forearms on the ground on either side of your body. Drive your hips up toward the ceiling so your body forms a straight line from your ankles to shoulders. Your toes, but not your entire feet, should be on the ground. Make sure your elbows are aligned below your shoulders and are about shoulder-width apart. If flat palms bother your wrists, clasp your hands together in front of you.

As you inhale, feel the expansion of your belly. As you exhale, contract your muscles to pull your navel up toward your spine.

Make sure you exhale through pursed lips, making that "S" or "Ph" sound to activate the core muscles. Engage your core not only by using your exhalation, but also by squeezing every muscle in your body that you can find in your legs and glutes (buttocks) as well. Hold for ten seconds and then release.

Mastering this will lead to a greater internal understanding and relationship between the targeted muscles and your brain. This is your gateway to begin to experience the magic in your muscles. Everyone who has ever worked with me knows it is a blessing to feel that magic. That means you are able to do the work, and your muscles are capable of activating.

4. "Feel It & Fire It Up"—Move the Body

What is It?

"Feel It & Fire It Up" is a YES! Body technique that fosters a deep understanding between your muscles and your brain. 80 percent of your muscles are voluntary muscles, meaning that you have control over their movements. To exercise that control, you must gain an internal connection with each muscle group within your body. It is like building an internal computer system, creating the necessary wiring, data, and connections that create a complex network and store the memory of each muscle movement.

The YES! Body System ignites your internal power through movement, awareness, and breath.

How to Do It

This process is designed to activate every muscle in your body. It is simple, but daily commitment is essential.

- Choose a muscle group (back, chest, legs, arms, core) to target.

- Choose an exercise that uses the selected muscle group as a primary mover or the main muscle that will activate during movement. Consider a plank, sit up, squat, lunge (*front, back, side*), chest press, lateral pull, push-up, etc.

- Inhale as you prepare for each movement and slowly exhale as you slowly execute each movement. Connect your breath with each movement.

- Do each selected exercise slowly and experience the sheer magic of negatives—feeling the muscle fibers as they are lengthened slowly under load.

- With each movement, practice deep diaphragmatic/pursed-lipped breathing, inhaling through your nose in preparation of the movement, and exhaling through your mouth during execution.

- Hold each position for three to five seconds with an isometric hold, where muscle tension is created without contracting the muscle. This hold creates a foundation of functional strength and is a wonderful way to really feel each muscle group at a deeper level. Isometrics help train the nervous system to coordinate with and fire the muscles in the proper timing to hold a specific position.[41]

---

41 Amy Marturana Winderl, C.P.T, "What the Heck Are Isometric Exercises, Really?" Self. com, June 23, 2020, https://www.self.com/story/isometric-exercises.

Each variation in the position of the muscle during the selected exercise creates a new challenge.

Follow these steps and start to feel the magic in your muscles!

Making it Work

My journey into the world of fitness was based upon the Feel & Fire It Up method. I used this YES! Body method to discover my body's ability not only to do various exercises but to unleash its unlimited power source. I challenged and created a new relationship between my brain and my muscles by focusing on each movement with awareness and using focused breath. With each new discovery, I experienced the excitement about what was possible.

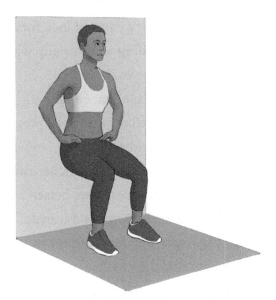

Wall-Sit

The Wall Sit

One such discovery involved the simple movement of the wall sit. Simply stand with your back against the wall, step your feet two feet away from the wall, and open your legs at about hip-distance apart. While keeping your shoulders against the wall, slowly and carefully lower your body until you are sitting in an imaginary chair.

Once seated, take slow, focused breaths and become keenly aware of everything you feel within the muscles and where you feel it. Every sensation is magic. Every sensation helps build the internal library you will use when doing any type of exercise in the future.

Find the Fun in Fitness

What if you could wake up every day and look forward to exercising? What if you felt something was missing when you were unable to exercise? That can be you!

Many of my participants experience that reality. I love that Linda, who had not exercised before joining the program and had several bad eating habits and health risk factors, now says she wants to exercise, enjoys walking, and very often exercises twice a day. Due to her new YES! Mindset, Linda describes herself as, "energetic, adventurous, and excited to see what my body can do." Linda began this process at age fifty-eight, and her journey continues.

Now is your time to find the exercise style that excites you—the style that makes you want to come back again. Lasting commitment to your fitness journey requires you to dedicate your brain and body. You can fire up that dedication even more when you allow yourself to try something new.

Try a piece of equipment, a new class, or an exercise you can do by yourself or with others. If you like walking, try a fabulous nature hike. The key is to stay committed to learning all that you are capable of. Step into your excellence and make a new challenge to find another level in your life.

The key is to Commit to Ten. If you commit to moving ten minutes daily and do it consistently, you will experience change. Most importantly, you will set your body on a steady track toward transformation. This type of transformational change will not only improve your physical health but also reinforce the components of the YES! Mindset.

Science Speaks

"Physical activity maintained throughout life is associated with lower incidence cancer, diabetes, and cardiovascular and coronary heart diseases. Recent studies suggest that physical exercise also protects against dementia."[42]

The YES! Take-Away: *It is never too late to find your fit—Commit to be Fit and nourish your brain and your body!*

---

42 L. Bherer, K. I. Erickson, and T. Liu-Ambrose. 2013. "A Review of the Effects of Physical Activity and Exercise on Cognitive and Brain Functions in Older Adults." *Journal of Aging Research:* 1.

CHAPTER 11

YES! LIFE VS. COMPARTMENT LIFE

You have done it! You've taken the basic steps to advance your personal journey. By realizing the importance of honoring the true you, finding those authentic aspects of your personality and your character that make you special and unique, you have taken a major step toward reaching any goal you set for yourself.

Now, you are ready to take the next step. Living the YES! Life requires a constant commitment to keep working toward your vision and expressing the authentic person you are.

All aspects of yourself require ongoing attention. For instance, we all have to constantly work on our character through reflection. Periodically ask yourself: Am I a compassionate, loving, kind, patient, and giving individual with self-control? Am I that person whose light shines bright on all those who come across my path?

You owe it to yourself to continue striving to become the best of you. When you do that, you will not only attract all those who walk in a similar light, you will also encourage others to strive to be the best of themselves.

Even though, at times, the discovery process might be quite painful as it takes you down roads filled with disappointments, negative thoughts, and old bad habits, it is an essential part of your journey and will set you on a pathway of endless wonder and life-altering possibilities—the pathway of hope.

Having traveled that pathway to achieve the YES! Mindset, you can now set your sights on fulfilling the purpose God has placed upon your life. You are now prepared to live as you were intended to live—moving out of internal blindness into your external, vibrant vision. Before you spring forward into the next phase of your YES! Journey, I want to leave you with one more vital piece of information.

The Power of Wholeness

It is essential that you recognize the difference between living the YES! Life as a whole, integrated being and living a compartmentalized life in separate "buckets" that do not connect with each other—or yourself.

So many of us live our lives as if we are multiple, separate people. We each live our career life, parental life, spouse life, friend life, all while trying to tend to our spiritual life, fitness life, nutrition life and time permitting, hobby life.

It is exhausting just thinking about all the hats we try to wear effectively and all of the balls we attempt to juggle simultaneously. We feverishly work on improving one area to the detriment of another.

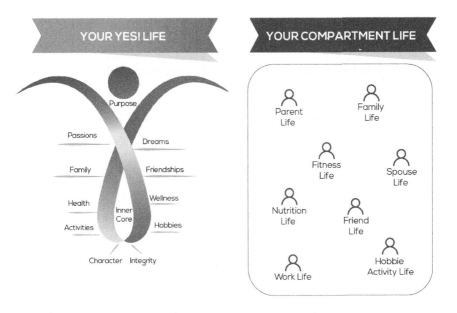

While you might experience fleeting or even lasting moments of success in one or more of your compartments, feelings of failure are often looming close by in others.

If your fitness life is together and you are working out as you have never done before, the nutrition life may fail you. Your body becomes fitter, but you become fatter. If your work life is great, your family life may be suffering. Relationships are strained, and happiness eludes you.

You can get to the point where you feel discouraged and incapable of meeting anyone else's needs, let alone your own. The "give-up" mentality is common in compartmentalized living. Feelings of failure can leave deep, lasting wounds, and if you're not careful, they can trap you within your separate parts.

I myself spent many years chasing individual buckets and experiencing the frustration that I could not "do it all." I didn't know how to live any differently. But another perk of growing older is that you also grow wiser.

Think of moments in your life when you have felt overwhelmed, under-appreciated, stressed, lost, defeated, and frustrated. Those emotions are often attached to the areas of your life that remain unfulfilled or unsustainable.

If you have ever just wanted to scream, "I just can't do this!" the good news is that you don't have to.

You have a choice to make. Like all the choices you made earlier in your life to do things that took you closer to your dreams or moved you closer to your pain center, the choice of how to live your life is yours. The choice has always been yours. You really can do George Jetson proud, and truly "get off this crazy thing!"

I love the point in *The Wizard of Oz* when Dorothy realized she could have gone home at any time simply by clicking together the heels of her beautiful ruby-red slippers. She had the power all along—and so do you.

> You have the power. So, what life do you choose? Compartment life or the YES! Life?

You have the power. So, what life do you choose? Compartment life or the YES! Life?

The Power of Connectivity

If you choose the YES! Life, congratulations! You can now live as one whole being, focused on a constant appreciation of your

Inner Core and all the factors that best represent who you truly are. This is exciting, as you were never designed to live a compartmentalized, disjointed life, wearing separate hats, changing yourself like a chameleon to meet different obligations while creating different relationships along the way.

Now you can just breathe and ready yourself for connective living.

Your commitment to live as one being is a commitment to learning how to unite your YES! Mindset with your brain-body connection and with your Age-Defying Life framework. The YES! Life recognizes that you will always need to balance all the things that make you uniquely you and leave behind the things that don't.

I mentioned in an earlier chapter that you are as unique as a snowflake: precious and rare. But when you try to live only one piece of your life at a time, you become fragmented and incapable of finding internal peace.

The YES! Life brings a sense of inner peace and connectivity by requiring you to make all your decisions from the inside out. You learn to operate at all times within the tenets of your Inner Core, supported by your continuous work to shape yourself as a person of integrity and great moral character. When all your actions spring from your Inner Core, they will naturally be connected and connective, not fragmented and compartmentalized.

You will also continually work to be of service to your health, to your family, to your faith, to your friends, as well as your passions, loves, interests. As you step with purpose, with faith, and with truth, you will find that all steps will lead to the life of your dreams.

Reflect Before Acting

To remain in balance and achieve that inner peace that rests within the YES! Life, always ask the following questions before you move into action:

1. What does my Inner Core tell me?

2. Are there core values or moral principles that can guide me?

3. Does this opportunity, decision, relationship, etc., nourish my true authentic self? (Remember: When you nurture your Inner Core, all elements of your life will continue to blossom.)

4. Will it allow me to live up to my highest standards?

5. What are the consequences of my action or my decision?

> Remember:
> When you nurture your Inner Core, all elements of your life will continue to blossom.

Simply taking a moment to ask yourself these key questions will unlock your ability to make decisions that are in line with your true needs and true desires. The YES! Mindset is not about agreeing to everything. It is about allowing yourself to express your true being, which also sometimes includes discerning when to say no.

Let your inner voice be a reflection of that YES! Mindset, so all decisions advance the values of love, peace, goodness, kindness, faithfulness, patience, and compassion. Each decision you make within those values will elevate the health of your brain, your body, and your beliefs.

The chart says it all: A life of confusion versus a life of purpose; a life of fear, frustration, and failure versus a life of love, understanding, and compassion. There is nothing more inspiring than a person who has the veil removed from their eyes and can now see their path with clarity, optimism, and an endless sense of wonder and excitement.

> Are you ready to step into your excellence? Are you ready to live according to your Inner Core, the authentic you?

Is that you? Are you ready to step into your excellence? Are you ready to live according to your Inner Core, the authentic you?

The YES! Take-Away: *The YES! Life may sound like a dream, but if you are willing to step into your greatness, do the work, follow the path, and commit to be committed, it is yours!*

CHAPTER 12

FROM PAIN TO PROSPERITY—LIVING THE YES! SYSTEM AND LOVING LIFE!

Well, we've made it through our journey together. Now is the glorious time to step into your true desires. Now is the moment to realize that moving forward means understanding all of what makes each of us unique. "All" includes, as stated in a Clint Eastwood movie, The Good, the Bad, and the Ugly. The YES! Journey honors all facets of our authentic selves.

I walked the Yo-Yo path for more years than I like to count, but I took the steps to break out of the negative mental habits that were holding me back and step into my YES! Mindset. I processed my pain. I stopped ignoring it and burying it so deep that I deceived myself into thinking it had no impact on my life.

No matter where you stand on your own path through life, it's never too late to transform your journey into something bold and new. I've given you plenty of examples to prove that. What are you waiting for?

COMMIT

Now, when I think back on painful experiences, I focus on the positive lessons I learned and bathe in the positive emotions that flow from my personal growth. That power is inside you as well.

I own the choices that I have made and will continue to make, and I now have power over the internal voices that used to spit fire at me and attempt to derail my successes.

Most importantly, I took time to discover and gain a deeper understanding of my Inner Core—the authentic me. I know my loves, my passions, my gifts, and my talents, and I know what is most important in my life. I work every day to achieve my God-given purpose with truth and faith for the future.

Will you join me?

You can work within your own newfound YES! Mindset, committing yourself to creating a positivity zone where optimism, inspiration, passion, and compassion can thrive. That is the YES! Life, and it is a place of internal peace, where compassion and understanding for self and others can rest within the center of your words, thoughts, and deeds.

DO

> We all do this life only once—there's no time to live small.

With the YES! Mindset comes the responsibility to take action toward fulfilling your life purpose and reaching your true desires. To Do, you must first jump into the ADL—the Age-Defying Life—and be prepared to commit to age with grace and excellence. Be age-honest and constantly challenge yourself to enhance your brain-body connection as well as your positive belief system.

We all do this life only once—there's no time to live small.

Because you are one entity—brain, body, and spirit—your journey toward the completion of any goal must include a commitment to advancing your health, top-down, inside-out. When you explore your core, you reacquaint yourself with each of your body parts, creating that mind-muscle relationship and embarking on honest, connective living.

The H2H or Healthy Healing Habits will enhance your brain-body connectivity, your Vitality Pump (deep diaphragmatic breathing), and your Fueling and Fitness Habits. The H2H will have you sleeping more and stressing less. You will be on the road to a healthier you with more energy and vitality than you could have ever imagined.

LIVE

Our greatest adventures lie within each of us. We all have the opportunity to take our dreams, hopes, desires and determination and create a life of endless possibilities. I can say that in my journey to manifest possibilities into reality, I have experienced both happiness and sadness, ups and downs, triumphs and defeats, and the many faces of pain.

Each moment of your life is like that snowflake. It is rare, one-of-a-kind, never to happen again. Melted away, it could represent a moment of consequence or a missed opportunity for growth. It could have been a transformational thought, missed through the distractions of meaninglessness. That sounds harsh, but its truth could never be more certain. The land of the living focuses on the beauty in this world and thrives on the loves and passions we choose.

I chose a YES! Life. What do you choose?

Here in the land of the living, be present. Don't give way to living in past thoughts or future worry. Discover how to keep only those things in your life that advance your YES! Mindset, and discard the "bad apples" that don't.

I loved the scene in *Willy Wonka and the Chocolate Factory* where Violet Beauregarde didn't follow the rules and was squished like a blueberry. Like a bad fruit, she was discarded and prevented from derailing everyone else's journey.

Will you discard your "bad apples"?

Produce the best fruits with your labor by remaining dedicated and consistent to your journey. Every day is a new day of self-correction and new opportunities. And finally, persevere. There will be storms and setbacks and challenges, and that is OK! It is called life, and unpredictable changes and events will happen. This is the time for you, the Relentless Warrior, to arise and, as my grandfather would say, "know the measure of your soul."

With your new YES! Mindset, you will find your ability to withstand life's challenges and to step up to your excellence is greatly enhanced. You are powerful, and it is time to step into those Super-Power Adjectives you claimed earlier in this book.

The rest is up to you.

But you don't have to travel alone. Brain science says that emotional support "is a significant protective factor with respect to cognitive aging." We need each other to cheer, to encourage, to help, and to dance in shared triumph when we reach goals and experience success.

Science Speaks

According to data from the MacArthur Studies of Successful Aging, levels of emotional support are related to better cognition in men and women. This longitudinal study indicated that baseline emotional support also serves as a significant protective factor with respect to cognitive aging.[43]

I would love for you to join my YES! Tribe, my supportive Facebook group, as we elevate the principles of "COMMIT. DO. LIVE." If not, find a friend, a family member, or a church or community group to join you as you embark on what will be an amazing YES! Journey.

The doors are wide open, and the possibilities that lie ahead are vast. What will you make of them?

---

43 T.E. Seeman, T.M. Lusign, M. Albert, and L. Berkman, "Social Relationships, Social Support, and Patterns of Cognitive Aging in Healthy, High-Functioning Older Adults: MacArthur Studies of Successful Aging." *Health Psychology*, 2001, 251.

YES!
COMMIT DO LIVE

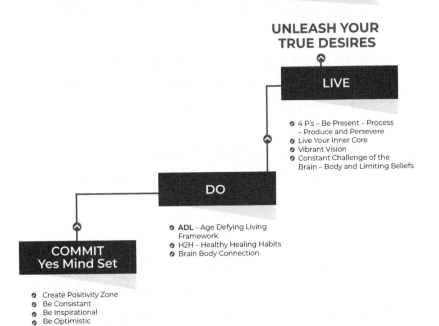

**UNLEASH YOUR
TRUE DESIRES**

LIVE

- 4 P's – Be Present – Process – Produce and Persevere
- Live Your Inner Core
- Vibrant Vision
- Constant Challenge of the Brain – Body and Limiting Beliefs

DO

- **ADL** – Age Defying Living Framework
- **H2H** – Healthy Healing Habits
- Brain Body Connection

COMMIT
Yes Mind Set

- Create Positivity Zone
- Be Consistant
- Be Inspirational
- Be Optimistic
- Thrive in Compassionate Thoughts – Words – Deeds
- Build Your Character

THANK YOU

I would like to thank my family for their ongoing support during this book-writing process, which often interfered with family time. I love you guys!

I thank Bernadette Fausto, Ph.D. (Cognitive Gerontologist); Karen S. Basedow, MS, RD, CDE (RWJ Barnabas Health; Dr. Jason Levine; and Dr. Terrance L. Baker for taking the time to read my book in advance of publication.

I also thank my "Jointly Fit Together " crew for being wonderful colleagues and friends.

I thank my "Fit Mind, Fit Body" crew and all my church fitness class family for being dedicated participants—and a special thank you to those who allowed me to interview them for this book. I am so appreciative.

I thank my RWJ Beth Israel Medical Center family for our ongoing relationship and my Beth Israel class members, who will always hold a special place in my heart.

I thank my colleagues at the Rutgers Aging & Brain Health Alliance for immersing me in the land of neuroscience—a new passion unleashed.

I thank all my training clients over the years. You all helped me to create the material for this book.

And I would like to give a special thank-you to Nicole Gebhardt of Niche Pressworks for helping me to launch my vision!!

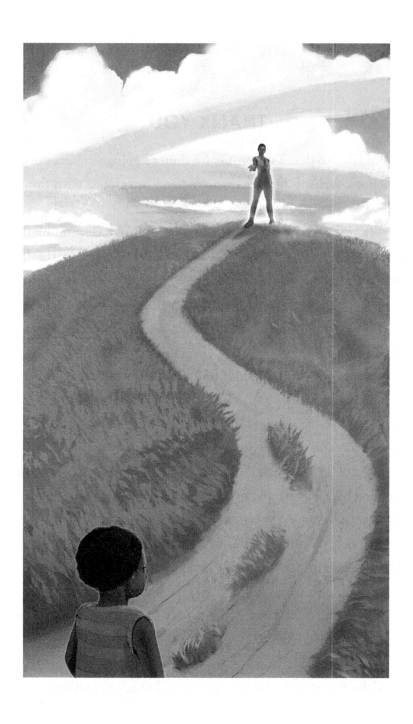

ABOUT THE AUTHOR

Lisa Charles is a federal prosecutor turned singer/actress, wellness expert, certified health coach/consultant, and an acclaimed speaker. She is the fitness/wellness research coordinator for the Rutgers University Aging & Brain Health Alliance, CEO of Embrace Your Fitness, LLC, and the author of *YES! COMMIT. DO. LIVE.*

She successfully directed her struggle with temporary vocal loss into personal growth by shedding 77 pounds without dieting. This ignited her zeal for fitness, cemented her understanding of the brain-body connection, and prompted her to delve into the process of creating a life based on passion.

Today, Lisa empowers individuals to let go of their limiting beliefs, embrace who they truly are, and breakthrough any age-limiting barriers by allowing them to experience wellness from her top/down, inside/out approach. Her strategies are centered on transformational techniques within and outside the Fitness industry that produce tangible, lasting results.

She lives in New Jersey with her husband.

You will:

- Sleep More,
- Breathe Deeply,
- De-Stress,
- Eat Healthily, and
- Move the Body to advance your Balance, Coordination, and Strength!

For healthy tips and free downloads, join Lisa's email list at: www.YesCoachLisa.com/resources

Join the YES! Coach at: www.facebook.com/yescoachlisa and learn how to live an Age-Defying Life!

It's a Wellness Revolution!

YES! COMMIT. DO. LIVE.

Social Media

Linkedin: www.linkedin.com/in/embraceyourfitness

Instagram: www.instagram.com/lisaembracefitness

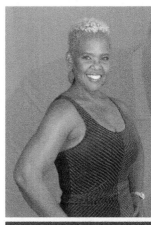

LISA
CHARLES
HEALTH COACH AND TRANSFORMATIONAL TRAINER

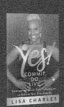

Lisa has served as the Fitness/Wellness Research Coordinator for the Rutgers University Aging & Brain Health Alliance. She is an Author – Health & Wellness Speaker and Consultant – Certified Health Coach – Transformational Trainer. She is also the CEO of Embrace Your Fitness, LLC, a health and wellness consultancy. Lisa is the creator of "Yes! Commit Do Live" a Book and program that teaches individuals how to live an 'Age Defying Life' while attaining Brain/Body Connectivity. It helps people break through any age limiting barriers to experience wellness from the top/ down — inside out, providing a pathway towards achieving optimum brain health. It is a Wellness Revolution!

SPEAKING TOPIC

- Commit. Do. Live. – How to turn true desires into real results
- Brain-Body Fit – Top/Down – Inside/Out Fitness
- The 1-2-3's of Exercise made Fun
- Breathe Yourself to Health
- Create Your Wellness Revolution

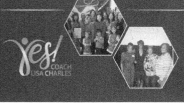

yes! COACH LISA CHARLES

www.yescoachlisa.com

lisa@yescoachlisa.com

https://bookme.name/yescoachlisa

Made in the USA
Middletown, DE
23 September 2021